Art Therapy and Creative Aging

W9-BLY-914

Art Therapy and Creative Aging offers an integrated perspective on engaging with older people through the arts. Drawing from the author's clinical, research, and teaching experiences, the book explores how arts engagement can intertwine with and support healthy aging.

This book combines analysis of current development theory, existing research on creative programs with elders, and case examples of therapeutic experience to critically examine ageism and demonstrate how art therapy and creative aging approaches can harness our knowledge of the cognitive and emotional development of older adults. Chapters cover consideration of generational, cultural, and historical factors; the creative, cognitive and emotional developmental components of aging; arts and art therapy techniques and methods with older adults with differing needs; and examples of best practices.

Creative arts therapists, creative aging professionals, and students who seek foundational concepts and ideas for arts practice with older people will find this book instrumental in developing effective ways of using the arts to promote health and well-being and inspire engagement with this often-underserved population.

Raquel Chapin Stephenson, PhD, ATR-BC, LCAT is an associate professor and art therapy program coordinator at Lesley University.

Art Therapy and Creative Aging

Reclaiming Elderhood, Health and Wellbeing

Raquel Chapin Stephenson

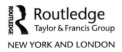
Routledge
Taylor & Francis Group

NEW YORK AND LONDON

First published 2021
by Routledge
605 Third Avenue, New York, NY 10158

and by Routledge
2 Park Square, Milton Park, Abingdon, Oxon, OX14 4RN

Routledge is an imprint of the Taylor & Francis Group, an informa business

© 2021 Taylor & Francis

Library of Congress Cataloging-in-Publication Data
A catalog record for this title has been requested

ISBN: 978-0-367-37025-1 (hbk)
ISBN: 978-0-367-36225-6 (pbk)
ISBN: 978-0-429-35275-1 (ebk)

Typeset in Times New Roman
by MPS Limited, Dehradun

This book is dedicated to my teachers, most notably those whose stories appear in this book.

Contents

xii *Contents*

List of Illustrations

Figures

Tables

Foreword

When Raquel Chapin Stephenson invited me to introduce the book you are about to read, my first reaction was to suggest that, at 84, I could hardly be objective about anything involving getting older. She told me that her primary message was an upbeat one, and that my usual perspective would be compatible with what she had written. Indeed, she was right.

As I reflected on almost 60 years of doing and writing about art therapy with individuals of all ages and conditions, I know that one of my core beliefs is the power of positive expectations about every human being's capacities. Having genuine faith in each individual's creative potential is absolutely essential to facilitating anyone's development through the arts, regardless of age or situation. If anything, this conviction has only grown stronger over time.

I am honestly not sure how or when I first learned this vital truth, but I suspect it was the repeated experience of discovering creative gifts hidden within so many of the children with whom I began my art therapy career in 1963. From the start these youngsters, despite their discouraging diagnostic labels and genuine deficits, taught me – by their uniquely personal inventiveness with art materials – that everyone carries within themselves the ability to create. I was lucky to learn this lesson, which may have been especially powerful because my teachers were children usually viewed with pessimism. That prejudice was as pervasive then as ageism often is now.

Fortunately, there is considerable evidence that positive expectations, regardless of the source, can and do lead to successful outcomes (Rosenthal & Jacobson, 1968). Although the original research was done in the sixties, the phenomenon has since been studied in a wide variety of settings with diverse populations, and it has been demonstrated repeatedly that what is popularly known as a "self fulfilling prophecy" is in fact true. Called "the Pygmalion effect," I believe it is also applicable to expectations about people's ability to blossom creatively.

The book you are about to read is infused with the author's passionate desire to improve the lives of those who live longer through meaningful arts engagement. Raquel Stephenson's approach is based on her deep and abiding faith in human potential. Because the unquestionable sincerity of her belief shines throughout between the lines of her text, reading this volume is far more than informational and informative; it is also inspirational.

Since I and my cohort are living longer lives than previous generations, the rapidly expanding number of elders is a fact. Given the paucity of literature on art therapy with older adults, there is no question that there is an urgent need for guidance in this area. This book therefore is a most timely gift. The reader is also fortunate that the author is as well prepared as any to take us on a tour of this particular territory.

It is immensely reassuring that, after 20 years of extensive experience with many different kinds of arts programs for older adults, Raquel Stephenson is firmly secure in her belief that all elders are capable of enhancing their lives through arts engagement, regardless of their particular physical or mental conditions. Her enthusiasm is palpable, which no doubt accounts for much of her success with those she has served.

She has worked with old folks in a wide variety of settings, including psychiatric and medical hospitals, rehabilitation facilities, community centers, and more. She has led groups in locations representing both the best and the worst in spaces for creating, from well-equipped art studios to shared kitchens or basements. She has done art therapy with elders experiencing Alzheimer's disease and other dementias confined to nursing homes, as well as high-functioning older adults living independently and attending an open studio.

In fact, Dr. Stephenson's journey itself, which she describes in some detail, is quite instructive. The reader will learn about the evolution of the author's ideas and attitudes about art therapy with older adults as she encountered new and challenging experiences in the course of her career. The arc of this narrative will no doubt change in the future as it has so far, offering a useful model of lifelong professional learning.

It is understandable, especially given the challenges of this population, that some become wedded to a particularly effective methodology that is then elaborated over time. Such a solution is tempting in its stability and predictability. There is tremendous security in knowing, and a great deal of anxiety in uncertainty. Being able to sit with not knowing takes courage, a quality that is never claimed by the author, but was apparent to this reader throughout the book.

Following the organic development of her ideas is therefore fascinating, because rather than assuming she has found the answers, Dr. Stephenson has been an explorer, continually in search of greater understanding. As her universe of practice expanded and changed, so did her thinking. Like her optimism about elders' creative potential, I find the story of the author's own growth to be similarly hopeful. Her way of thinking about her work is, like her doing of that work, curious and open, modifying as she goes along. Clearly, her belief in the power of the arts to enhance and enrich the lives of even the most diminished elders is the foundation for her enthusiastic promotion of such programs.

But how, I wondered, is it possible for an arts provider who has spent so many years entering the world of those whose capacities have diminished, to maintain such consistent optimism? It can happen only when the perception is, as I believe is true for Stephenson, thoroughly honest and open-eyed. It is this quality that makes her recommendations so credible, because they are based on the reality of old age, with all its painful challenges.

Getting older is neither easy nor fun. Romanticizing old age is dishonest. Although many have found ways to enjoy and value this time of life, there is also general agreement that the "golden years" turn out to be more tarnished than shiny. Even without major disease or disability, many aspects of normal aging really do make it more difficult to function. These include sensory losses – in vision, hearing, touch, smell, and taste. Even those who remain active notice changes that gradually limit coordination, balance, and mobility. And the natural lessening of cognitive capacities makes it harder to think or plan or execute as quickly and easily as in the past.

Dr. Stephenson's approach to these impediments is refreshingly clear-eyed and realistic. Far from denying their existence, she acknowledges them and is empathic about their impact on the individuals whose stories she tells. She addresses deficits in a matter of fact way, offering pragmatic solutions and numerous examples of trial-and-error problem solving. What shines through, when she is dealing with such difficulties, is a flexibility and open-mindedness about the uniqueness of each situation as a new puzzle to be solved.

There is, in other words, a felicitous combination of clarity about problems and optimism about potentials. These issues become real as we hear stories about people who come alive for the reader. We meet three women interviewed by the author who attended an open studio, each discovering a new identity as an artist. We get to know them intimately through her eyes, as she strives constantly to see their worlds and their creative work through theirs. Most striking is that her initial expectation of what they could teach her about art in old age was dramatically modified by what she actually learned.

Later, we meet others, some of whom the author saw in individual art therapy, for whom the challenges of creating were more formidable. What is clear is that these elders are viewed as respected collaborators with the art therapist, as she helps them to access their strengths in order to express themselves. Many of these stories are poignant, because of the degree of disability with which some were coping. The reader will find their narratives deeply moving, as person and practitioner work together to find a way for each to express their authenticity. While their artistic voices range from mute to articulate, the honoring of their humanity is consistent.

This book is full of such close-ups, heartening narratives about individuals who found their voices on the nonverbal avenue of art. In addition, the author also offers us a panoramic view of the territory of art for elders. Because of the exponential growth in numbers living longer lives, art programs have sprung up in numerous settings, serving not only those requiring treatment, but also those wishing to fill increased leisure time with meaningful activity.

The many and varied programs described by Stephenson serve an expanding group of older individuals, and they do so with a rapidly diversifying group of practitioners. Just as the activities described in this book are carried out with a growing range of participants in an increasingly wide variety of settings, so they are being offered by an ever growing variety of providers. Their ranks include not only art therapists, but also teaching artists as well as doctors, nurses, social workers, medical students, caregivers, and eager volunteers from all walks of life.

The notion that it is both possible and desirable to make creative activities available to more older adults is based on a growing body of evidence that "arts engagement improves health and well-being." This is not only the subtitle of this book; it is, I believe, its most urgent message. Like Viktor Lowenfeld (1952, 1957), who taught art educators that access to creative activity should be the right of every child no matter their abilities, Stephenson's zeal is passionate.

Reading this book often reminded me of Lowenfeld's words about the importance of making art available to all:

> "Wherever there is a spark of human spirit – no matter how dim it may be – it is our sacred responsibility as humans, teachers, and educators to fan it into whatever flame it conceivably may develop. ... We are all by nature more or less endowed with intrinsic qualities, and no one has the right to draw a demarcation line which divides human beings into those who should receive all possible attention in their development and those who are not worth all our efforts. One of these intrinsic qualities is that every human being is endowed with a creative spirit."
>
> (1957, p. 430)

In addition to the moral imperative of Lowenfeld's manifesto about every human being's creative rights, making the arts available to more older adults has huge secondary gains, saving medical dollars by improving health and wellness. The reader is introduced to the impressive findings of researchers like Gene Cohen, about how arts activities for elders dramatically improve health in measurable ways, like reducing the number of hospital and doctor visits or the frequency of falls (Cohen et al., 2006, 2007). These studies were based on groups led, not by art therapists but by artists and teachers, and are intimately related to a contemporary revolution in health care heartily embraced by Dr. Stephenson.

This radical transformation of the arts provider landscape has brought people other than arts therapists into contact with a great variety of vulnerable populations, including older adults. One of the most helpful parts of this book is the author's clarification of the movement known as "creative aging" (Hanna et al., 2015). It is similar to the "arts in health care" or "arts in medicine" movement, in that its practitioners include physicians, teaching artists, arts educators, performers, and others, as well as creative arts therapists. In fact, as the author explains, the two developments are related both historically and conceptually.

This is understandably a complicated issue for many art therapists, but since it is happening so rapidly and in so many places serving older adults, learning about it from an art therapy educator will be incredibly helpful for readers. Stephenson's enthusiastic description of the expanding realm of arts activities for elders illuminates its richness and beauty. She discusses the intersectional questions it raises, while rejoicing in its potential to enhance even more lives.

Given this openness, it will come as no surprise that her perspective includes the values of looking at as well as doing art, exemplified in the many museum-based programs around the country. The author opens the door as well to other art forms – music, movement, drama, poetry, any and all creative activities that can enhance and enrich people's lives. In valuing the contributions of many different arts providers, her open-minded perspective opens the windows of potential gain that much wider, letting in even more sunshine.

I am reminded of the film, "Alive Inside," (Rossato-Bennett, 2014) that tells the story of an idea born in the mind of Dan Cohen, a social worker visiting nursing homes. His inspired thought was simple – provide residents with headphones through which they can hear the music of their youth. The results were so exciting and dramatic that he and the film's director both created foundations to spread the word about what they had discovered. Watching these depressed elders coping with dementia brighten incredibly as they listen is truly thrilling. Happily, a recent large-scale study found measurable evidence of the effectiveness of the "Music & Memory" program for participants: statistically significant reductions in psychotropic medicines and improved behaviors (Bakerjian et al., 2020).

There's yet another kind of openness in this book that readers will discover. It is the honest recognition that, while products, exhibits, and performances may be the visible outcome of arts activities, much of their therapeutic benefit lies in the social and emotional pleasures of being with others and sharing their artwork with friends and family. The bonds formed by arts group members, revealed when they gather even during a leader's absence, are a reminder that these groups are an important part of each other's support system. Loneliness is a growing problem for many isolated older adults. It is refreshing to be reminded that, like the art process itself, these interpersonal connections are a major source of the life-enhancing aspects of such activities.

Similarly, it is wonderful to be reminded of one of the many reasons that making art is such a source of joy: the sensory pleasure of working with materials, the fascination of manipulating colors and textures, the sheer fun of exploring possibilities and different media. At the same time, the author acknowledges the frequent need for the art therapist's "third hand" (Kramer, 1986). When working with those whose capacities are waning, the therapist's task is to provide what's missing to make creation possible, making this work inherently collaborative, even when it happens in a group.

Given her wealth of experience, Raquel Chapin Stephenson has learned a great deal about procedures that work when offering art to older adults. In this book she generously shares what she has discovered with the reader, spelling out ways of shaping the space, selecting materials, and presenting tasks. She offers thoughts about structuring the session, creating continuity, and providing closure. That she has learned from helping so many different kinds of older adults in such diverse settings makes her advice all the more credible. These nuggets of wisdom about her lived experience in this domain are a gold mine of information for anyone wanting to lead art groups for elders.

As a reader, I am grateful to the author for her generosity, her openness, her optimism, and most of all for her emphasis on joy. All too often art therapists are taught to focus on goals that meet the requirements of treatment planning, whether they are positive like improved self-esteem or reparative like reduced anxiety. But the honest truth is that all human beings, especially as we age, long mainly for happiness with a grin, for the experience of being "alive inside," of feeling joy.

Engaging in art activities that are novel and stimulating in old age has an added benefit, regardless of the particular knowledge or skill involved. It has to do with the power of learning something new at the very time that one is facing both the decline of the body and the approach of dying. Many years ago when I was about to retire from practice, I read an article that made a huge impact on me, probably because it expressed truths I had yet to acknowledge. I was looking forward to having more freedom to travel, and this article spoke about its deeper value in the context of aging:

"Travel allows one to feel new when it is no longer possible to feel young. Every day, just by being alive, kids have experiences from which they grow and learn, while the rest of us have to pursue the new, struggle against inertia and push ourselves to keep growing, a task that gets more difficult as we become more set in our ways. But when we take a trip and enter unfamiliar settings, we reconnect with our childish sense of wonder and discovery, and we discover an unexpected bonus: The clock slows down and life seems to expand."
(Pogrebin, 1996, p. 33)

The author of that article was 50 when she wrote it, and I was 60 when I read it. I was still able to learn tap dancing at 62 and to travel to many continents for over 20 years. The message, however, remains valid regardless of chronological age or condition. If we replace the idea of "travel" with "creating art" it becomes clear that what is most exciting and enlivening and often thrilling is that making art allows one to feel new when it is no longer possible to feel young.

As Pogrebin suggested, when we travel to an unfamiliar place we are able to reconnect with our childish sense of wonder and discovery while seeing, smelling, and hearing the richness of another culture. Anyone who has experienced the excitement of playing with materials, with ideas, and producing something that never before existed in the world, knows that making art brings a similar kind of aliveness. When one is engrossed in creating, it is absolutely true that, as in her description of travel, the clock slows down and life seems to expand.

This, I believe, encapsulates the contribution of this book. The author's message to the reader is a reminder of the value of being open to any and all possibilities for enhancing old age through arts engagement. This includes welcoming many options – about the where, the how, and the who of making the arts available to elders, in a way that recognizes their assets as well as their liabilities, and does so respectfully, kindly, compassionately.

As for "reclaiming elderhood," the other part of the author's message, there is surely benefit in viewing old age as bringing potential growth as well as inevitable decline. Whether everyone achieves wisdom is debatable, but there is no question that having lived longer and seen much change over time results in a more informed perspective. It may also bring a more nuanced understanding of the world and of how human beings function, permitting more effective navigation of complex interpersonal situations. It is also true that getting older allows one to speak more candidly, and to be less concerned about what others might think. There is an increased freedom to explore new realms and ideas, unconstrained by prior roles and responsibilities. Without question, there are gains as well as losses in the aging process.

Raquel Chapin Stephenson has given us a wonderfully informative guide to all that arts engagement can bring to older adults. The reader will be introduced to experiences as rich in thoughtfulness as they are in detail. As we take in her learnings and her teachings, we discover that it is indeed possible for those in the golden years to shine, to feel more alive, and through creating, to feel joy.

Judith A. Rubin
PhD, ATR-BC, HLM

References

Bakerjian, D., Bettega, K., Cachu, A., Azzis, L., & Taylor, S. (2020). The impact of music and memory on resident level outcomes in California nursing homes. *The Journal of Post-Acute and Long-Term Care Medicine*, *21*(8), 1045–1050.

Cohen, G. D., Perlstein, S., Chapline, J., Kelly, J., Firth, K. M., & Simmens, S. (2006). The impact of professionally conducted cultural programs on the physical health, mental health, and social functioning of older adults. *The Gerontologist*, *46*(6), 726–734.

Cohen, G., Perlstein, S., Chapline, J., Kelly, J., Firth, K., & Simmens, S. (2007). The impact of professionally conducted cultural programs on the physical health, mental health, and social functioning of older adults: 2-Year results. *Journal of Aging, Humanities and the Arts*, *1*, 5–22.

Hanna, G.H., Noelker, L.S., & Bienvenu, B. (2015). The arts, health, and aging in America: 2005–2015. *The Gerontologist*, *55*(2), 271–277.

Kramer, E. (1986). The art therapist's third hand: Reflections on art, art therapy, and society at large. *American Journal of Art Therapy*, *24*(3), 71–86.

Lowenfeld, V. (1952). *The Nature of Creative Activity*, 2nd ed. London: Routledge and Kegan Paul.

Lowenfeld, V. (1957). *Creative and Mental Growth*, 3rd ed. New York: Macmillan.

Pogrebin, L. C. (1996, April 21). And Miles to Go. *New York Times, Section 5*, 33.

Rosenthal, R., & Jacobson, L. (1966). Teachers' expectancies: Determinants of pupils' IQ gains. *Psychological Reports*, *19*(1), 115–118.

Rosenthal, R., & Jacobson, L. (1968). *Pygmalion in the classroom: Teacher expectation and pupils' intellectual development*. New York: Holt, Rinehart & Winston.

Rossato-Bennett, M., McDougald, A., Scully, R. K., Cohen, D., Sacks, O., McFerrin, B., Shur, I., ... & MVD Visual (Firm). (2014). Alive inside.

Preface

Art Therapy and Creative Aging is about reframing our understanding of elderhood and, specifically, how engagement in the arts is life-enhancing, joy-inducing, and promotes well-being. The goal of this book is to inspire the reader to engage in, create, and support creative arts therapy programs for older adults in order to foster the health, well-being, and actualization of a growing, important, and at times marginalized population, while being accessible and fun to read.

If you have ever visited assisted living facilities, you may have noticed they all have a similar look. You walk in through a grand entrance, where you encounter a large bouquet of fresh flowers on a table in the foyer, plush furniture, a library, and maybe a piano. Brochures and websites for potential residents list the many activities available, including arts programs, for residents. My experience working with some of these organizations, however, revealed an unnerving contradiction. While they are keen on making a good first impression, and acknowledge the value of arts programs – including art therapists – in practice, they use them as a marketing piece. In practice, very little art therapy is offered, often only a few hours per month. The situation is similar in nursing homes.

My experience with these facilities led me to conclude that in order to provide meaningful creative arts therapy to older adults, to build it as a field of study, and contribute to the body of knowledge that supports it, I needed to become part of the small but enthusiastic community of artists, art educators, and art therapists who dedicate at least part of their careers to using the arts to better the lives of elders. I have had the joy of working with several such innovative organizations, and they have informed and inspired the course of my career.

I was fortunate to have a close relationship with my grandparents. Much of my childhood was spent with them, and we shared deeply in each other's lives. They lived active and healthy lives into their 80s, but when my grandfather became ill and was unable to maintain the active life he had once enjoyed, he became unhappy. Although he said he felt useless, I didn't see him that way. To me, he was a wise, loving, and interesting man who still had much to offer. I wondered if there was a way to re-engage him. I wondered if art or music might help to lift his depression or if it might help other older adults who were also struggling. Because of this experience and my deeply held belief that art can be a powerful, therapeutic asset in life, I returned to school to become an art therapist. I hoped that through art I could help older adults cope with illness, loss, or periods of transition.

In my 20 years in this field, I have met many older men and women who showed me that maintaining engagement in old age is indeed possible, and so, too, is re-engagement in the face of loss or change. One woman I worked with, who began making art at age 87, described her experience as exploring a part of herself she never knew was there. Individuals who became blind late in life have used art as a way to cope with their circumstance, developing an enhanced sense of touch and spatial awareness through art – skills that were vital to maintaining their independence. And I am constantly amazed at how the art-making process opens new pathways of communication for those who have lost their ability to communicate verbally because of Alzheimer's disease yet are desperate to connect. Art has been a powerful tool in facilitating their expression.

Recently, while teaching in China, I was introduced as having a career spanning 30 years. I corrected the person introducing me, in part because I don't deserve those ten unearned years but also because I wasn't quite ready to age so quickly! My colleague was quick to point out that seniority and age are supremely valued in China, so the introduction was meant to be a compliment.

In my midlife, what I often don't consider, is how with each passing day, month, and year, I become more experienced as a human being, with the ability to draw from an ever-growing cache of experiences that help to guide and inform me in big and small ways.

While writing this book, I learned how to kayak in whitewater, a sport I had wanted to try for decades. Each day on the river I learn new skills to maneuver my little plastic boat through the rapids from one eddy to the next. It is thrilling to be a beginner again! I didn't expect to embark on learning a technically and physically challenging sport again, but it has made me feel alive, challenged, empowered, excited, motivated, joyful, and happy.

I have witnessed incredible vitality in people who continue to learn until the day they die. I have worked with people even in their 100s who take risks in art-making and other areas of their life. While recent literature on art therapy with older people lean into a more positive view of aging, such as being empowered (Partridge, 2019), there remains limited research in art therapy and creative aging with older people. Filling this gap, in some modest way, has been a motivating factor for my research and subsequently writing *Art Therapy and Creative Aging* – wishing to share my research findings and field experience with elders who exemplify growth and lifelong learning.

I cannot say that I don't fear aging in some way. The past is known, but the future is uncertain. What if I am no longer able to remember the information I have so painstakingly learned throughout my life? What if I lose physical functioning, or it declines to a point where I can't do the things that make me happy? At the same time, perhaps I will get better at some of the things that I struggle with now, such as being fully present with myself or having space and time to connect with others. I hear from older friends that they are becoming more selective in how they spend their time and less concerned about what other people think. I'm looking forward to that.

I am aware that, of course, many challenges become more intense with age. My own grandfather, faced with several debilitating illnesses in his last decade, used to say, "Aging isn't for the faint-hearted." My grandmother, who experienced much joy in her life, would probably not have said her last few months were joyful, as her health declined. Each person I have worked with as an art therapist has confronted age-related challenges, crushing losses, and fear. But most were not without hope, an eye toward the future, and that something special that makes working with older people so captivating. Somehow, I become a better version of myself alongside the golden cast of their beautiful souls.

Reference

Partridge, E. (2019). *Art therapy with older adults: Connected and empowered.* Philadelphia: Jessica Kingsley Publishers.

Acknowledgments

Writing this book was many years in the making, during which great amount of learning, listening, trying, watching, filtering, applying, and wondering changed me and how I understand the work that I do. While these pages are the result of two decades of work and learning, the final, heaving effort required to produce it in this written form also did not happen alone. My clients, students, colleagues, and teachers have been instrumental in my learning each step of the way, and especially the NYU CATS student interns brought joy and creativity to the work – together we learned so much. I am grateful to Lesley University for affording me the gift of time to see this work through, and especially to my colleagues who graciously filled the void while I was on sabbatical.

I would like to specifically acknowledge Ikuko Acosta, Elizabeth Hartowicz, Vivien Marcow Speiser and Eha Rüütel for their enduring mentorship and meaningful collaboration with me in projects included in this book. Additionally, I wish to thank Rebecca DiSunno, Karen Estrella, Jeanne Geers, Eileen McGann, Nisha Sajnani, and Janine Tursini for generously taking a peek and offering advice at a pivotal point in idea development. Sue Motulsky and Donna San Antonio were steady sounding boards as I sorted through ideas. Stephanie Beukema helped me to keep the goal in sight, even when it was just an idea with a plan, and to pay attention to the paving stones guiding my path. Maddie Gerig Shelly expertly gathered current research on numerous topics. The keen editing eye of Ed Levy transformed this pile of words into something readable. Routledge editorial dream team Amanda Devine and Grace McDonnell were a pleasure to work with. And, a heartfelt thank you to Judy Rubin, a foundational teacher of mine from the very beginning, for generously writing the foreword to this book.

Although no longer in the living world, I leaned heavily on three people from beginning to end: my grandparents, who nourished me with empathy, generosity, and grounding, and my mother, whose tenacity and endurance is evidenced by this book. My extended family cheered me on from near and far, celebrating milestones with me along the way – especially my sister

Andrea who gifted me with lobster and champagne when the first draft was complete. I am eternally grateful to my immediate family who gently endured living through this journey by my side – my husband Ed's steadying touch kept the ship from capsizing, and my son, Will, kept the wind in my sails, reminding me each day, "You've got this, Mom!"

1   Introduction

I was very close to my grandparents. I loved being around them and their friends, so it felt natural for me to choose to work with older adults. I value older people, and I saw a huge need for services for them. Most of my classmates wanted to work with children, but none, other than me, chose to work with older people. My grandmother, again and again, encouraged me to focus my work on children. She would say, "Raquel, why would you want to work with older people? Why not work with children whose lives are just beginning and where you could make a real difference?" Although I had taken her advice on so many other occasions, clearly I did not follow it this time. I wondered, Does she really believe that a younger life is more valuable than an older one? Had she bought in to our society's bias against age? I wish I had asked her these questions at the time.

My career as an art therapist has been so joyful – well beyond the enjoyment I anticipated at the outset of graduate school. When my clients experience comfort and joy, I understand and know this by a kind of natural reciprocity. This is at the root of my fascination and delight in working with this population. One of my main goals now as a teacher has been to share the joy I feel in working with elders in hopes of encouraging new therapists to choose to work with them as well. Although there are a limited number of available jobs and a small number of people trained to do this work, there is a great need for it.

The subtitle of this book, *Reclaiming Elderhood, Health and Well-being* is intended to reframe the way the latter part of life is viewed. In many ways, American society views elderhood as a long extension of adulthood, without accepting it as its own developmental time and stage. Geriatricians Bill Thomas (2014) and Louise Aronson (2019) speak of reclaiming elderhood by understanding older adults from their unique perspective and assets; elderhood, in their view, is the third act following childhood and adulthood. Aging is not only about biological decline. That's part of it, of course, but it is also about growth. Older adults possess so many attributes that are overlooked and misunderstood and many that have not even been discovered.

Purpose of the Book

This book is for creative arts therapists, creative aging professionals, and students who seek foundational concepts and ideas for practice. Although it contains many practical tips drawn from my experience in the field, it is not a how-to guide for initiating art or art therapy activities with elders or people with dementia. Rather, its aim is to inspire the application of arts engagement with older people in the broadest way possible. *Art Therapy and Creative Aging* offers an integrated perspective, drawing on the ideas of creative aging and current knowledge of the cognitive and emotional development of older adulthood, a unique stage of life.

I hope it will inspire older people, their families, and all stakeholders in the care of elders, to imagine new ways to engage them in arts for the betterment of their health and well-being.

My Limitations

I am a middle-class, middle-aged, white American woman, originally from the Midwest, and the approach to creative engagement presented in this book is inevitably influenced by my lived experience. My professional experience has been primarily on the East Coast of the United States and in large urban and suburban cities. In my community-based work, the majority of participants, although they represent each socioeconomic class and diverse cultural backgrounds, have also been white and of European descent. They were able to participate in these community-based programs because they possessed the financial means, mobility, proximity, or caregiver support.

At the inpatient geriatric psychiatry hospital unit where I also worked, my patients were more diverse racially, culturally, medically, and in terms of age. Many did not have the financial or social resources to soften the ravages of mental or dementing illness. I recognize the wide disparities in how Black and indigenous people, all people of color, and other marginalized older people fare in many areas, including health, longevity, and access and quality of care, to name a few. The Covid-19 pandemic has only widened the chasm, evidenced by a higher rate of infection and death.

Learning from this book needs to be extracted with a critical lens and applied with awareness to people across race, ethnicity, gender, age, and religious and sexual orientation.

My Inspiration

I can't even begin to count how many conversations I've had with colleagues, friends, and family members who sink into worry about preserving functioning, beauty, and health. Rarely do we discuss the emerging freedoms gained as we age. And yet, many older people have told me they are happier later in life than they were as a younger person.

People like Adeena, who, after retiring, had a tremendous passion for making art and devoted most of her time and energy to it! Or Marina, who, despite coping with significant arthritic pain each and every day, came to the studio to make art in community. Their openness to learning something new about themselves left its mark on the way I see aging and my vision of how the arts can improve lives in a multitude of ways.

Older people have inspired me. I have heard from them the many interesting experiences they have had in life, and they have shared so much wisdom and experience. But what has been most meaningful for me is the resilience displayed by those elders who have endured immense loss and change.

A Few Words About Terms

Most often, I refer to the people in this book as "older people." The term describes a segment of the population who are more advanced in their stage of development relative to others while at the same time implicitly acknowledging that all of us are getting older, not just adults. At other times, I will refer to these same people as "elders" as a means of respect and valuing the unique stage of life called "elderhood." The terms used in this book for the consumers of arts engagement include "artist," "participant," and "client." I have been careful to name a person as a client only when they have been referred to clinical treatment.

The terms used to describe the arts engagement practitioner in this book are more specific, at times, referring to the professional "art therapist," "creative arts therapist," or "teaching artist." At other times, I use "arts in health practitioner" to refer to the wider field of those who work in the arts with older people, including, but not limited to, therapists and teaching artists.

State of Aging in America

There is much that concerns me about growing old in the United States. We haven't yet figured out how to embrace the aging of our society, to see it as a gift that could benefit us all. Instead, the conversation is focused on the global decline in births and increase in lifespan. We hear that dementia is on the rise and that the baby boomers will drain Social Security as they reach retirement age en masse. Beauty products and pharmaceuticals are marketed to our fear of aging and promise to roll back time. (As if we could!) We are looking at aging all wrong.

Rather than see older people as targets for youth-promoting, turn-back-time products and fear-mongering about all that will sag, wrinkle, and break as we age, we would do far better to celebrate lived experience.

We should truly honor our elders not only because they are intrinsically worthy of respect but also because we value those qualities that improve and expand with age – qualities like wisdom, creativity, and problem solving, to name a few. If we reframe what it means to grow old from this perspective, we can redesign our interaction with aging – our own, that of our loved ones, and the aging of our society.

What are the ingredients of a joyful elderhood? As I write this, I am years from being considered an elder, but I have been fortunate to know many older people who are joyful in their later life. Can we reframe our perspective on aging, shifting negative ageist stereotypes to recognition of new and different attributes and opportunities that are – or could be – gained in later life?

Research and innovative practice help us to understand how old age is different than ageist rhetoric has led us to believe. We know more about the aging brain and its potential and unique capacity. There are countless opportunities for elders to reframe their own vision and engage with life. It has prompted a new way of understanding aging – not as a stage of decline and decrepitude but one of hope, joy, and possibility.

Health and Well-Being Are Human Rights

The health and well-being of older people are human rights. We need to better understand the lived experience of all communities of older people and make policy changes that serve their real needs. Our current dominant biomedical paradigm of care supersedes the choice of the older person when that paradigm conflicts with their lived experience. Moving toward relational and contextual paradigms of care, where the perspective and experience of the older person is centered and valued, will align medical care and social services to a more ethical continuum of care and toward, as Bill Thomas (2014) proposes, "a life worth living."

Understanding how life is valued from an older person's perspective has led to a reevaluation and recalibration of the measures we use. Aronson (2019) paints her experience as a geriatrician with broad strokes of science and the humanities to offer a rich, nuanced perspective of aging that is full of "joy, wonder, frustration, outrage and hope about old age, medicine and American life" (p. xiii). Gwande (2014) suggests that we shift from simply prolonging life at all costs to valuing quality of life, yielding a perspective in which an older person is empowered to assert their own definition of a life worth living. Thomas (2014) emphasizes how human beings cooperate with others to exist across the lifespan. "We grow, mature, and then age, and at every point along this journey, our well-being is tightly interwoven with that of those around us. Aging changes the nature, not the fact, of our reliance on others. Aging is the ultimate team sport" (p. 69). Finally, Thomas identifies three main factors that determine well-being: strength, purpose, and belonging. Strength is needed in order to live life on our own terms, purpose is needed to have a reason to live, and belonging is needed because it is essential to have relationships and to be included in community.

Of course, growing old is not without its perils, especially for those who are poor or in poor health. But it is important to not ignore the unique attributes that older adults possess and to use them to build bridges of connection and health engagement. Among these attributes are increased creativity, increased ability for risk-taking and spontaneity, a greater capacity for solving complex problems, and a greater ability to navigate complicated interpersonal, social, and politically charged situations.

In the Pages Ahead

Art Therapy and Creative Aging offers an overview of the ways arts engagement is an effective path toward health, well-being, and joy in later life. While arts engagement is hardly new, we are learning more about how our capacity for creativity expands with age, as shown in the stories of Rose, Adeena, and Marcia in chapter 2 and in the research on creativity in chapter 3. Chapter 4 presents a framework that readers can use to explore their own generational perspective in relation to someone from another generation. Chapters 5–9 offer details of creative arts in practice with older people, such as the intersections of care available, from the expressive therapies to arts in health (chapter 5), the goals of arts engagement (chapter 6), the structure of the arts encounter (chapter 7), and a discussion of art materials in chapter 8. Lastly, chapter 9 explores art-making with people who have dementia.

Art experiences can help people realign their sense of self to embrace the wisdom that comes with the changes in thinking, feeling, and behaving that occur in later life. Art, for many people, is a transcendent experience, one that allows for the past, present, and future to co-exist at once. Through engagement in the arts, powerful and meaningful emotional content can be expressed, examined, and recollected with changed understanding or purpose.

Arts engagement fosters joy, celebrates life, and promotes health and well-being in a variety of ways, and contributes to a life worth living. This book presents concepts, research, and theories that support this claim and methods for how to implement it.

References

Aronson, L. (2019). *Elderhood: Redefining aging, transforming medicine, reimagining life*. New York: Bloomsbury Publishing Inc.

Gwande, A. (2014). *Being mortal: Medicine and what matters in the end*. New York: Metropolitan Books.

Thomas, B. (2014). *Second wind: Navigating the passage to a slower, deeper, and more connected life*. New York: Simon and Schuster.

2   A Portrait of Three Older Artists

Rose, Adeena, and Marcia are elders I had the good fortune to interview for my doctoral research about the experience of people who choose to make art later in life. They shared with me many aspects of their lives, and their stories, combined with those of countless older people with whom I have worked, formed my understanding of how the arts enhance well-being and soften the aging process.

Rose

> *"Art has been an enabler for me. I feel very secure in the fact that I am an artist … it gives me a feeling of total confidence." – Rose*

During our first introduction, in a telephone interview, Rose would not reveal her age but confirmed that she was older than 65.

> I don't tell my age. And that's not because of me but because of other people. I have some companions who would be reluctant to go out with me knowing that I am that many years older than they, and so I don't tell my age. But mostly it's because of the artwork, because I don't want anyone looking at something and saying, "that's beautiful, pretty good, considering her age." My age has nothing to do with that any more than my age has anything to do with anything else I've found.

Rose was a warm, kind woman, short in stature, with smooth, short gray hair. When we first met, she greeted me with "Hello, dear" at the door of her apartment. Her eyes were bright and always connected with mine, conveying a sense of deep commitment to what she was telling me and ensuring that I connected with what she was saying. She walked slowly, with a slight limp, but never complained about her arthritic pain.

Born and raised in New York City, Rose had lived alone in her apartment since her husband died 20 years earlier after a long illness. The apartment was high up in the building, open to bright light that flooded in through large windows. The living room was neat and clean, with decorative rugs covering the tile floor, artwork (hers and others') filling the walls, with well-cared-for mid-century style furniture. A television and stereo sat discretely in a large built-in cabinet along the center wall. For our first interview, she prepared a tuna sandwich with lemonade for me. We shared a little about our common interest in art, and she said that she was happy that I was interested in what she had to say. She told me about her family. She has a son and grandchildren who live in another state. Active in the community, she attended a variety of classes and taught writing and art appreciation.

Rose didn't begin to paint until age 40. Until then, her only creative activity, as she described it, was sewing or fashion sketching, as she was raised in a family of seamstresses and clothing designers. She said as a young woman she felt worthless and that her sole purpose was to be a wife and a mother. At one point, a friend introduced her to painting, which opened her eyes to her hidden talent but also to her unique voice. She began to feel her opinions mattered. From there, she began taking art classes, and art became an important part of her life.

Rose began making art by taking classes to broaden her skills and confidence but eventually realized she preferred to work alone, with the exception of occasionally attending my open art studio. While she enjoyed learning from an art instructor, she did not feel any pressure to adopt their style or technique. She was careful about receiving criticism and said she preferred it come from those who she thought were better artists than she was – she did not particularly like critiques from "any old body, smart as they may be." She showed her work in a gallery, which led to showings at two more galleries, and felt good about the acclaim she received from having her work noticed and exhibited.

The main themes that emerged in my interviews with Rose were:

- The value and importance to her of being an artist
- How it has been a means for her to connect to others as well as across the generations
- The influence of aging on her art, and of art-making on the aging process

Through her art, Rose told me, she is trying to communicate "whatever is good about me":

> Through my art, I am expressing what I am. It's not just something that I do because I enjoy it. Art has been very much an enabler for me. I feel very secure in the fact that I am an artist. I know where I am. I know my level. I think I have done some things that are good, and that makes me feel good.

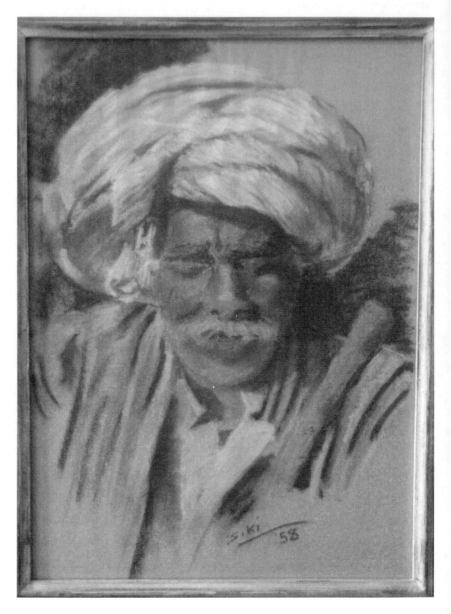

Figure 2.1 Bedouin Man.

One of her earlier works, *Bedouin Man* (Figure 2.1, Bedouin Man), drawn in 1958, is an 11 × 14-inch pastel based on a black and white photograph. Rose explains:

> *Bedouin Man* was an exercise in using pastels. The teacher would bring in black and white photographs and give them to us to develop

in color. Wonderful exercise! He handed me that one, and I worked on it, and as it developed, it was great. I brought it home one night, and my husband had already gone to bed, but I said to him, "Can you wake up long enough to look at something?"... He followed me into the living room. I stood it up on the bookcase, and he said, "You are never, never going to sell that one. That one is mine. That is the way I want to grow old! Look at the look in his eye." I enjoyed doing that.

This drawing was particularly important to Rose, and she spoke of it often, mostly because of the powerful connection her husband had with it; it was as if the drawing was a form of ongoing connection with him. But while he had remarked about the "look in the man's eye," Rose seemed more drawn to the powerful transformation that adding color had had on the image. The blue background is bold and commanding, offering a stark contrast to the subdued colors of the man and his clothing. This process of transforming an image from black and white to color was liberating for her, allowing her to use creative license to make the photograph into a drawing that was very much her own expression.

At the time of our first interview, Rose had stopped making art, stating that she had become frustrated with making art and was experiencing a "block":

> For several years, I would say at least 3 years, I have been living in a state of bitter frustration. I haven't been able to do anything artistically. I suppose I do some things, but I haven't been able to create a picture. If I get something started, I am unable to finish it. And the frustration is difficult.

Instead of making art during this period, Rose got a lot of satisfaction from teaching art-appreciation classes. She also began experimenting with creative writing. When I returned for our second interview, she showed me a pastel drawing entitled *Nighttime Beach Scene* (Figure 2.2, Nighttime Beach Scene) she had recently created that pulled her out of her slump.

> I started out with a very pale sketch of this photograph of a beach in the morning. Then it went on from there. I'm not sure what it says – nothing special, but these things have certain meanings. I think it has something to do with my feeling about water. If I feel troubled, I know that the sound of the surf will have a calming influence. I'm not alone. I know other people who have this feeling, too. The sound of the ocean has that effect.

Figure 2.2 Nighttime Beach Scene.

Rose wondered aloud if our interviews had prompted her to begin working again. She felt satisfied by the drawing and immediately bought a frame for it and hung it in her apartment. Drawn quickly, at a community open studio art group, it has loose strokes and creates a soft, impressionistic feeling of serenity. Rose described looking at a photograph of a beach that served as a guide. She felt it was "very fresh and very current." I think that the abstract nature and freedom of the drawing might have loosened her up, allowing her to take the risk of making something in the midst of a creative block. What was most striking was how relieved she was. Being able to make art again was enormously empowering and showed her that she could overcome obstacles to achieve her goals. This loosening up, or movement toward abstraction, is also evident in her later work, when she again utilized this approach to overcome obstacles to making art.

As Rose talked about her creative process and her artwork, it became clear that for her, the wider context of being an artist in society, such as the sense of empowerment it brings, was of utmost importance. Being an artist made her feel she is "not totally useless":

Art has opened doors for me that have nothing to do with drawing and painting. It has given me the understanding that there is creativity in so many things, many ways to be creative." She said she felt confident when in the company of other artists. Before finding art, Rose said, she didn't value what she had to say. "Art has given me the confidence to talk to people because I know that, no matter what, there will be a level at which I can communicate. I know that the confidence, the self-confidence is there. Sometimes I have to push down the feelings of inadequacy. I actually have to say to myself, "No, that's not your opinion, that's your mother's opinion or your sister's or your aunt's or somebody's opinion. I wanted opinions, even if they were adverse, from people who were at least as good or much better than I. And there are many.

Rose found art served as a bridge to engage with people of any age. "It is wonderful talking to you," she told me, "because I could almost be your grandmother." Art is the great age equalizer, she said, and described how, as she grew older, she became more outgoing about meeting new people. She has also gained an important perspective: When you are young, she said, you want to be loved by all, but she knows now that is not how it works: "Now, I want to be respected, but not by everybody. I want to be respected by the people whom I respect. Art has done that for me."

She acknowledged that aging influenced her art but said that, conversely, art-making influenced her aging process:

I don't think I'm getting overly poetic about things, but the painting has grounded the aging, and the aging at the same time is grounding. I approach my aging without resentment. I feel as though I have delivered some kind of message. Something has made my years worth it ... I'm more able to face my age. The fact is, there are things that are good about aging once you accept yourself as the subject of aging.

Rose said that her approach to making art changed as she got older. She accepts that she is talented, but at the same time, "I don't feel that before I die I must turn out the great American masterpiece." It was, she told me, important to make art that was satisfying to her, not necessarily to the general public.

While she had a higher level of confidence, Rose's physical limitations, such as arthritis, at times prevented her from doing something she wanted to do. For example, she said that her arthritis didn't prevent her from holding the paintbrush, but it did affect the way she moved it.

After our interviews, Rose had surgery and was quite ill. Because her right arm was immobilized, with the encouragement of her son, who recognized the importance to her of making art, she began drawing and painting with her left, non-dominant hand. As a result, her work became

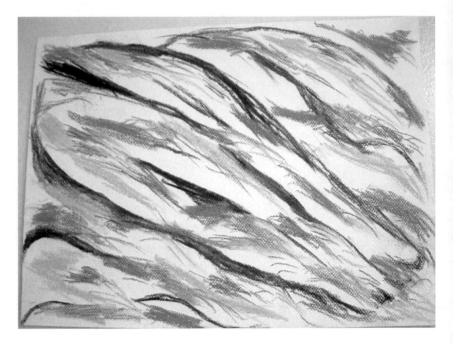

Figure 2.3 Racing Colors.

completely abstract – yet, she felt liberated by this change and empowered by her ability to work without the use of her right hand. This shift seemed reminiscent of her approach to creating *Nighttime Beach Scene*, which had released her from her creative slump. In this phase, she used playful stories to guide her work. For example, a pastel drawing *Racing Colors* (Figure 2.3 Racing Colors) depicts a story she invented about the primary colors (red, yellow, and blue) running across the page when suddenly black enters the picture and chases the colors back to the other side. Using a story to guide and structure her work was a new and creative approach that allowed her to continue her engagement in and enjoyment of making art.

Pictorially, *Racing Colors* is the most expressive, playful, and humorous of all her work I had seen. Despite persistent illness, Rose was able to create imaginative and expressive work, and most importantly, she was able to transcend her physical limitations to continue to express herself through art.

Adeena

> *"I feel that everybody is worth remembering, but particularly people whose lives have been really disrupted by war, or taken by war." –* Adeena

Adeena was a bright, energetic 79-year-old who was born and raised in England. Petite, with brown hair, she dressed with a flair for fashion. Often, she wore a bright red scarf in her hair with matching lipstick or a colorful vest or jacket with black pants. She spoke with a lot of intonation in her English-accented voice and was passionate and inquisitive. She also had a wry sense of humor. She walked quickly wherever she was headed and interacted with people with the same sense of urgency.

Our conversation touched on many topics, including:

- Her early life and later success as an artist
- The influence of WWII on her work
- The influence of aging on her art and of art on aging
- The meaning of her art
- Her thoughts on leaving a legacy

Adeena began by speaking about her childhood. During World War II, she was one of many children sent from London to the British country-side to protect them from the German bombing raids. During her short stay there, she became seriously ill with tuberculosis and was moved to a medical facility, where she remained until the end of the war. Her illness was very debilitating, and along with the separation from her family and fear of the war, it had a lasting impact on her.

As an adult, Adeena lived in New York. When we met, she had been divorced for more than 30 years and had two daughters and a grand-daughter who lived nearby. She had a close relationship with them but led an independent life. Until she retired in the early 1990s, she worked as a social worker with psychiatric patients.

Adeena explained that she wasn't encouraged to make art as a child, and her teachers even criticized her drawings. Although she had been creative in other ways, she didn't begin to make art until her retirement.

> I never got a chance to know how good I was at art as a child. I was nine when I was evacuated, and that lasted from 1939 to 1945. But the impact of that extended throughout my life, through immigra-tion, marriage, children, divorce, none of them conducive to making art. I went back to it very late, which is when I knew I was going to retire from my job. I had been making clothes and doing other things that fell into the realm of crafts but were better than crafts, really, and it's only since then that I've been doing what I think is "real art."

Adeena said that once she retired she felt free to make art. She said she felt this was true of many older people. "They've always been artists, but they – and especially women – haven't had the opportunity to follow it." Adeena frequently showed and sold her work and gained momentum and recognition in the few years I knew her. She recently sold out an exhibit, and a British gallery owner took one of her works to London to exhibit and drum up interest.

Working primarily in collage and assemblage, Adeena collected paper and objects and transformed them, collaging text, photos, and other textures. Once, she found a box on the street containing someone's personal documents, including a passport and photographs. She contacted the family and asked if they wanted the items. They didn't, so Adeena created a work of art in homage to this person she had never met. Making art about others from found stuff of theirs was based on a deep respect for that person, transforming them and, in a way, giving them a new life.

In speaking about one piece in which she used the bottoms of coffee bags with the names of the workers who inspected them, she said:

> I am always wanting to pay some kind of homage to workers, to ordinary people. My mother was a union person, and I am a union person. So, this to me is my homage to paper workers. I think that they are worth the paper. They're people who are invisible, and they're really very good people. When people ask me questions about what it means, I often say that it's something that is otherwise silent and I'm giving it a voice. They may not understand what I mean, but that's as far as I go because, you know, people have to find their own meaning.

For one coffee-bag piece, Adeena wrote a story on a scroll with the worker's logo from the bottom of the bag. She tucked the scroll in a little tube and hung it from the piece. "Nobody will ever read it, but I know it's there." She created several other art works in a series using the coffee bags. One *Coffee Bags* work (Figure 2.4 Coffee Bags) is like a tapestry of stamps amid squares of coffee-bag paper. The work is textural, with a protective medium covering and hardening the surface of the paper. The names of the workers on the stamps are small, and might go unnoticed as the centerpiece of the work, overpowered by larger stamps and black ink squares. Other examples of work from found materials are the *Art Students League* drawings (Figure 2.5 Art Students League), which began with a newsprint pad Adeena found in the garbage:

> Once at the Art Students League, I found a newsprint pad of drawings in the garbage. People tend to throw the practice stuff in the garbage. I thought the drawings were gorgeous, and I could not understand why this person threw them in the garbage. I would like to draw like that. So, I took them. Newsprint is not stable at all. It's very thin, and it tears easily. I charcoaled them more because they will fade and put used tissue over them to make them stronger, so that I could use them in pieces. Then I reduced and enlarged them and made them all different sizes. I've done a really nice job with some of them.

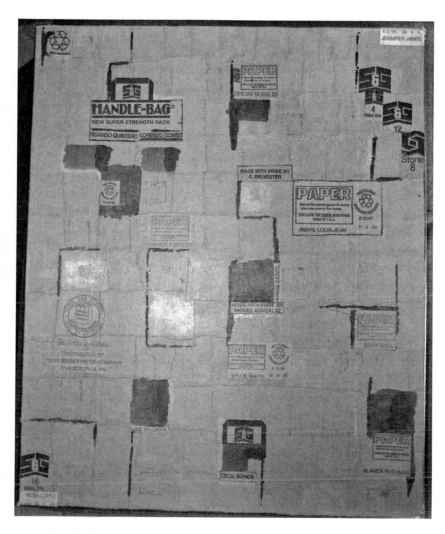

Figure 2.4 Coffee Bags.

Art Students League portrays three figures from the newsprint pad reinforced and collaged with others to create a dynamic composition of three figures in motion. Adeena added text that mentions Hitler at the very bottom and very top, inserting her own hand among these borrowed drawings in a subtle yet powerful way. Referring to the artist Robert Rauschenberg, Adeena said, "I am also compelled to rescue abandoned objects." Following our interviews, she created numerous pieces using these drawings, manipulating and transforming them even further.

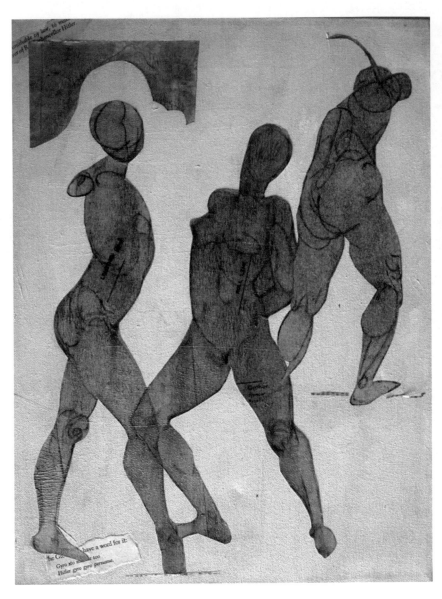

Figure 2.5 Art Students League.

As a child, Adeena made things from scraps of fabric. She recounted her beginnings assembling these scraps:

> During the war, we had shortages, and the shortage I experienced was of fabric because I liked to sew. I began to sew at 12. I put all my

creativity into the sewing because I had no other materials. I didn't even think of it as art, but I did have a reputation for sewing beautiful things using scraps. My mother and father brought home scraps from garment factories that were deployed to make uniforms. My aunt, who lived in the same house, worked for the queen's courtier and brought home better kinds of fabrics, but still scraps.

She remembers playing with found things, as there was no money for toys. "I think that was the beginning of what I do now," she said, "working with found things ... but which found things I work with is important. They are things I feel have some value."

Adeena came to realize that her interest in folded forms was unconscious and saw that it was like creating a book:

I think I've come to the stage of life where I feel I'm not going to have time to write what I wanted to write, and I don't even think I could. So I am basically putting my experience into objects that look like books. It seems more or less accidental, coming to this form, but it really wasn't.

Adeena's work is visual, textual, and textural, but it is not easily accessible. She is teasing her viewer to get a glimpse of a potent message, yet not revealing it in its entirety, such as in *Lysistrata* (Figure 2.6 Lysistrata). If a viewer is truly interested, she says, they will engage with the work and with the artist and might figure out what the work is about. She uses color and texture that is appealing but also evocative of potent emotions.

Adeena thinks her artwork draws people because of its content of wartime trauma. People come close to see what is written between the folds, yet it is concealed enough that it is impossible. "My instructor once said, 'You seduce and subvert,' and that is exactly what I'm doing. People look at these folded pieces, and inevitably they go up close to see what's in there."

Adeena acknowledged that her art seems very much related to her childhood experience, in particular to "loss, passion, and longing," as well as other losses during wartime, such as loss of time. She knows there is a correlation between reusing discarded materials, paying homage, and leaving her mark on this world.

Adeena made an important connection between trauma and artwork. As a child, she felt that she herself was "an abandoned object," and so making art that gives something a voice "arises from something in me that needs to be said."

She had recently moved, and made another interesting observation about death and dislocation.

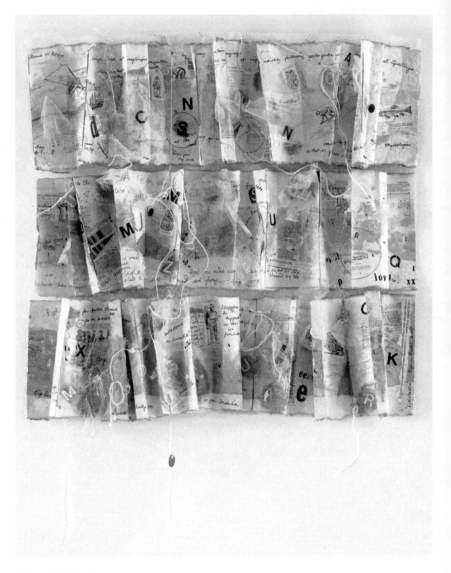

Figure 2.6 Lysistrata.

I think a lot more about my own death and about what I want to do before I die, and I feel some urgency about it, because I had to move [to another apartment], and that was in a way like the war all over again, being dislocated. In this building alone at least seven people I know have died since I moved in last August ... I certainly think about death now. How is it coming? When is it coming? How much will I be able to do? Why was my time taken away from me?

Adeena said that she was becoming more solitary, though others saw her as more gregarious:

> You're alone when you're an artist because you're thinking differently about everything you see. At first, this felt pretentious, but I'm feeling that way less and less. It's real, going back to what I said about the truth, – I'm trying to express the truth of who I am, of what concerns me.

Adeena viewed herself as a source of history, a vessel for preserving a legacy.

> I never valued what I had to offer before. Now I value it, and I want to say, "Look, you'd better look at this. It's not going to change anybody, but take a look." This is my work, and when my children come and clear up the apartment, maybe they will appreciate me. I know they appreciate me, but maybe they'll appreciate a side of me they didn't quite know was there.

Marcia

"I'm on a discovery mission, trying to fish for things." – Marcia

Marcia was a 90-year-old with loose, curly, gray hair that reflected her soft and easygoing demeanor. She walked and spoke slowly, which seemed to come out of a struggle to muster the energy and, at the same time, from careful consideration of her words and actions. She dressed casually in loose-fitting clothing and tennis shoes. During our interviews, Marcia led me around her apartment to show me various paintings. Her bedroom was her working studio, overtaken by a large, well used easel with a painting on it, overflowing boxes of acrylic paint tubes, and jars stuffed with brushes. Her double bed was placed at the center of the room, though it appeared the room was used more for painting than sleeping.

Marcia grew up on a farm in Vermont during the Great Depression. Her father was a woodworker from Romania and influenced her creative spirit, although as she described it, becoming an artist didn't occur to her until much later. Instead, she worked in the business world until her retirement. When she was in her thirties, she had her first exposure to an art class and later took night classes at the Brooklyn Museum of Arts School. However, she was primarily self-taught. In addition to painting throughout her adulthood, Marcia was an avid reader of art criticism; she was very clear about what she was doing and understood the art world.

Marcia touched on several main themes in our conversations.

- Her artistic process
- Her identity as an artist
- Her motivation to work
- Aging and the artistic process
- Art as a bridge to other people and interests

Marcia had been suffering from chronic fatigue syndrome that sapped her energy level, so it was hard for her to get around much. "I'm better now," she told me, "but for a number of years, it was like walking in mud. I couldn't seem to make headway. I painted, but it seemed like every painting was wrenched from me at great expense."

Marcia was a very prolific artist, and there were stacks and stacks of paintings in her apartment. We discussed many of her works, and I photographed some of them. She spoke of her work in terms of "periods," in particular her gray and white periods. Although a teacher once told her that at 40 years old, an artist's painting style is set, Marcia disagreed, noting that her style changed when she was 80.

Her process was to constantly mask out parts that she didn't like and add more. That is why at times one can see a ghostly halo of the paint beneath the veil. Marcia approached her work without a plan. She said she suspended preconceived notions of what a work would be about and just experienced the moment and the process. Rather than working from a sketch, she began right on the canvas with acrylic paint and let the image appear.

> When I approach a canvas, I have no idea where I'm going. There's nothing preconceived, and there's no inspiration. I just start making marks and shapes, and within those, I begin to pick things out …. I just fly without a compass. From moment to moment, I make decisions, change them, and then may go back to them. There's no agenda. Trying and retrying. I'm discovering myself. I'm on a discovery mission, trying to fish for things. I know there is a place where I can get images from, or I can get parts of images from and then supplement them from a more conscious part of the mind. If it doesn't fit in aesthetically or color-wise or form-wise in some way, then I'll eliminate, or my ideas will change along the way, which happens a lot … Sometimes something is lost in finishing it – I hate the word *finish*, but I use it – something is lost and something's gained in finishing.

Through making art, Marcia said she was discovering herself and her own agency: "I'm discovering that what makes me happy is that I feel I have a resource that can change, that's at my disposal if I work hard enough."

She said her artwork was about looking for metaphysical answers. She wondered if her gray period, which followed the paintings of black figures,

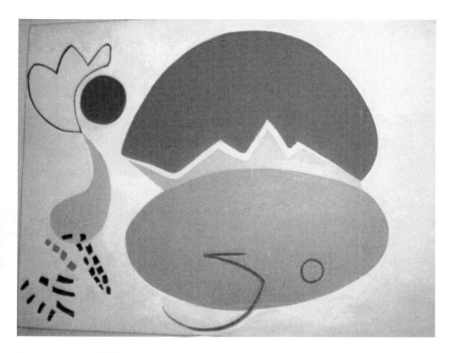

Figure 2.7 Untitled 1.

might be a reflection of both her sense of humor and her fear of death. During this period, she was interested in mysticism, and the paintings have more symbolism, such as in *Untitled 1* and *Untitled 2* (Figure 2.7 Untitled 1 and Figure 2.8 Untitled 2) – for example, Figure 2.7 is Shiva in the form of a woman, the pines of Rome, a Grecian column. A friend of hers had wondered if her gray period revealed a fear of death. Marcia felt that making that connection seemed too stereotypical:

> I don't know what it means. I call it *The Dream Body*. A friend saw one of my gray paintings and afterward saw one where the colors were bright and happy again. She called me and said, "I don't understand. These colorful ones are not your recent paintings, are they?" I said, "Yeah." She'd assumed that as you get older, you get so damned depressed, and that's what the gray paintings were about … The gray paintings for me weren't about depression. I had had a number of mystical experiences that intensely influenced the gray period.

Marcia said her process had not changed much over time, as she was always interested in flatness and working with different shapes. However, her new work was generally much larger, with a stark white background upon which she painted more angular, symbolic shapes, for example in

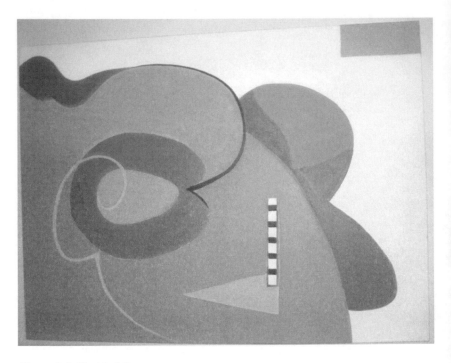

Figure 2.8 Untitled 2.

Untitled 3 (Figure 2.9 Untitled 3). The colors are more vibrant, and the shapes more complex. Overall, there is a bolder, more overt message being conveyed than in her previous work. She said:

> I think I'm about to go through a change. My paintings seemed holistic at one time; then they got into this fragmented stage and now I'm wondering if I can synthesize the holistic and the fragmented. I don't know. It'll come. I'm interested in both processes. I think this has something to do with my spiritual beliefs and feelings and how they've changed throughout my life ... I don't know whether I can control it or not but long before I change, I can feel things happening in my mind.

Marcia spoke about her identity as an artist and her motivation to work:

> For a long time, I didn't say I was an artist, a painter, or anything like that. In fact, years ago, the Women's Center had a symposium, and most of the women didn't come out and say they were artists. Thirty years ago, I certainly couldn't say "I'm an artist." Now I'm glad I have this identity as an artist. Maybe it's an ego boost, but as I age, I'm more ready to say that I am an artist.

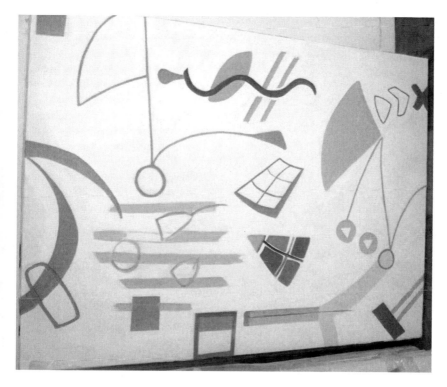

Figure 2.9 Untitled 3.

She believed that aging was easier because she's an artist:

> Art gives me a goal. I've something to do and something to reach for, which gives you more of a feeling of aliveness. I think I will always be working on some kind of project, doing something. I think being an artist has made aging easier – you are doing, you're planning, your mind is working, you're trying to link with something different and new and fresh ... I think it makes old age richer; as a result of painting, I have many interests. It's a bridge over to other things, a bridge to people, to other interests; it's enriching.

Concluding Thoughts

As younger women, Rose, Adeena, and Marcia each had an interest in art that returned and flourished as they aged. Initially, I was interested in learning about the difference in the themes and appearance of their art-work across the decades, but they were more interested in sharing with me the connection between aging and being an artist. Aging influenced their art, they told me, but more notably, being an artist made aging easier. How lucky was I to learn something far more valuable than what I set out to explore!

So many older people I have worked with reject the notion that they can make art and would never consider themselves artists. Yet, we now know much more about human development beyond childhood and adolescence than we used to and have a deeper understanding of development in old age: The mature mind is prime for creative and artistic endeavors. The old adage, "You can't teach an old dog new tricks," is simply wrong. In fact, older adults have a great capacity to learn new things, and their creative mind is primed for artistic activity, in which flexibility, risk, and imagination come into play.

3 The Reciprocal Influence of Art and Aging

Elders have demonstrated to me time and again how their creativity blossomed later in life. They are risk-takers with broad imagination and capacity for play, pushing their limits to learn and grow. This chapter will explore the creative potential of older adults, in particular that of Rose, Adeena, and Marcia – focusing on how aging influences art and art influences aging.

Developmental Influences on Making Art

Human development is a multifaceted phenomenon. The cognitive or personality development of a person involves the interrelation of cognitive functioning, autonomy, personality, and well-being; health; genetics; and biological processes. One way to understand human development is to adopt a "life course" perspective as proposed by Stowe and Cooney (2015), in which lifelong developmental processes and the arc of change and continuity are needed. A dynamic life course perspective considers lifelong development, history, and relationships. The unique life journeys of Rose, Adeena, and Marcia point to the complexity of decoding the influences of aging. Similarly, as proposed in Diehl and Wahl's (2020) lifespan developmental perspective, each stage of development is connected and equally important, changing in reaction to the interplay between biology and culture. Diehl and Wahl (2020) propose a "triple interaction" contextual approach to understanding lifespan development, whereby understanding the social-physical-technological context and the historical-cultural context of a person's life reveals how these components are in dynamic relation with one another.

The stories of Rose, Adeena, and Marcia support a variety of theories proposing that, from a developmental standpoint, creativity expands with age (Lindauer et al., 1997; Reed, 2005). Reed (2005) found that older artists felt more creative as they age. Investigating the self-perceived fluctuations in 21 artists' creativity between age 53 and 75, Reed compared earlier and later artwork and creative process changes, noting an increase in creativity felt by artists as they mature. Other themes that emerged as valuable to the artists were: lifelong expression continuity; life experience contributing to ingrained work patterns and experimental ability; compensation for changing physical and environmental factors; integration of life experiences; and creative motivation.

It has also been suggested that how a person behaves in old age is a continuation of how they behaved throughout life (Atchley, 1999); therefore, in part because of their lifelong patterns of behavior and wisdom gained from experience (Atchley, 1999; Cohen, 2005), these three women enjoyed multiple benefits through their involvement in the arts. Whether or not art itself was a lifelong pursuit, their level of engagement in creative activities throughout their lives established the pattern for their continued engagement in old age, despite its many challenges.

The theory of continuity and adaptation posits that a person's behavioral pattern continues throughout their life. Atchley (1999) outlines three continuity components: internal, external, and adaptive. Adaptive continuity features pathways in which a person continually adjusts to everyday situations. Atchley argues that while these coping strategies evolve and perfect over time, people generally use the same strategies throughout adulthood. According to Atchley, functional ability is the center of adult development. By middle age, most adults have strong ideas about their adaptive strengths and weaknesses and make choices that they see as leading to their strengths and minimizing their weaknesses.

Each of these women had in fact identified as "creative" throughout most of their lives, and by middle adulthood, all but Adeena had begun to engage in some art-making. This interest continues and has gained in importance – perhaps, as Atchley suggests, because as we age, we continue to involve ourselves in activities that enhance our strengths while minimizing our weaknesses. These adaptive strategies, built on continuity, helped them cope with disruptions like retirement, relocation, loss, and illness, providing a solid and stable form of continuity that helped them through a host of challenges.

While these women spoke of their interest in connecting with younger generations and demonstrated a certain level of wisdom, the bulk of their experience seems to fall outside of the Eriksonian model of looking back in order to face death (Erikson, 1959). Rather, these women were living in the moment, enjoying life, and in many ways looking forward and expanding their experience. This is not to say that they did not acknowledge or expect their own death. According to Erikson's stage theory (1959), each of these women was in the eighth stage of her life when I interviewed them, engaged in the struggle between ego integrity and despair. Each reflected back on her life, having felt satisfied by the good, and coming to terms with the bad. This struggle, according to Erikson, is the last step that each must pass through successfully in order to be ready to die, potentially becoming wise along the way. In light of the findings of my study, however, the Eriksonian model did not fully explain the developmental achievements of these women. Beyond merely looking back and preparing themselves for death, the three women in this study were vibrant women who, for the most part, were engaged in social and community endeavors that broadened their lives rather than simplified them.

Comparing the lives of these women to the Eriksonian model (1959), the increased feeling of kinship toward new generations and the desire to leave a legacy would fit squarely in the work of midlife, while reviewing one's life and accepting death would be that of the end of life. Likewise, Butler (1963) expands the idea that older adults naturally reflect back upon life, and that this review might take the form of storytelling, scrapbooking, art-making, or performance, the types of activities art therapy and creative aging engage older adults in. Cohen (2005) also contends that older adults reflect back on life, but adds that there is also celebration and continuation of life – a movement forward. In certain ways, each of these women was reflecting upon her life, and for some, like Adeena, it appears loudly in the artwork. Given the notion of life review, the life histories of these women also serve as a source of inspiration and material for their artwork. Drawing a conclusion that artwork that incorporates historical elements of their lives is evidence of life review might be too broad a generalization; yet, it may be considered a possibility.

Maslow (1968) suggests that individuals strive for self-actualization, the ultimate goal of human development. Assuming their more basic needs are met, then Rose, Adeena, and Marcia were presumably seeking a heightened level of satisfaction and wisdom. Each showed aspects of attained wisdom, as described by Baltes et al. (1992) and as expressed in their art-making. In particular, Rose felt very satisfied when she made a picture that she liked; Adeena felt satisfaction in her identity as an artist and in gaining recognition through prizes, awards, exhibitions, and the sale of her artwork. Marica reflected heightened wisdom in her later work and her ability to tap more deeply into her spiritual beliefs and aesthetic aptitude.

The experiences of these women suggest that making art contributes to "gerotranscendent" behavior, defined (Tornstam, 2005) as a transition from a materialistic and rationalistic perspective to a more cosmic and transcendent view of life accompanying the process of aging. While Tornstam suggests that the movement toward gerotranscendence happens naturally with age, these women showed that being an artist fosters this movement, as it gave them skills, strengths, and benefits in multiple areas that contend with the challenges of aging.

Understanding the dynamics of human development in old age from Tornstam's (2005) concept of gerotranscendence offers art therapists a solid and flexible developmental perspective from which aging might be understood. Building upon Erikson's stage theory, the theory of gerotranscendence moves beyond Western concepts of aging by drawing from

Eastern philosophies. It also opens up the developmental struggles in old age to include continued growth and maturation. Erikson's (1959) stage theory looks back upon one's life in old age in the eighth and final stage: Integrity vs. Despair; reintegrating those past experiences leads to wisdom (Erikson & Erikson, 1997). Tornstam's theory of gerotranscendence widens the possibility that while older adults do indeed look back and review their lives, they also continue to look forward. In this way, as Tornstam suggests, older adults develop new connections with both past and present. They envision themselves as part of a larger universe, or a move toward altruism. The continued movement toward self-actualization and wisdom, as noted by Tornstam, is evidenced by the experiences of Rose, Adeena, and Marcia. In this way, drawing from Tornstam's offerings of continued growth and development, art therapists might employ art-making as a means to foster such growth and movement toward gerotranscendence. Particular elements of Tornstam's theory are evident in the experiences of these women. There is a lessening of the fear of death and, concurrently, a greater interest in and appreciation of future and past generations. They saw themselves linked to a continuum of history rather than an individual mark in time.

Rose and Adeena both acknowledged that they have a great interest in sharing their experiences with following generations. It might be interesting to note again here that Marcia, who did not mention this desire, is the only of the three without children and grandchildren. And yet, Marcia's use of her art to transcend her illness has been especially notable. Her motivation to make art was more powerful than the physical limitations imposed by her illness, and she continued to paint prolifically when she was unable to do much else. She said that her need to make art forced her out of bed each day.

The women also expressed how they noticed the little things in life when they were older women. Although Adeena called dying "an insult," these women directly or indirectly also said they were more accepting of death. In addition, each mentioned that she had less need to be with others and has become more selective of whom she spent time with, which according to Tornstam's theory of gerotranscencence (2005), is a component of social transcendence. They noted that they were less worried about their physical appearance as they grew older. Tornstam (2005) categorized this as body transcendence – a greater acceptance of age-related physical changes and the ability to continue with many activities despite limitations.

To varying degrees, these women agreed that their art and aging processes were related. Old age also gave them more freedom, including time to spend on making art and the emotional or psychic space to explore their past, present, and future with a softened fear of criticism or failure.

Developmental Changes to Creativity and the Creative Process

The notion of creativity has evolved over time, from Rank (1932) asserting that regulating sexual urges generates the desire to create, to Freud's conviction that creativity is a type of desire satisfaction (Freud, 1952), and Kris's (1952) exploring creativity in the preconscious mind. Winnicott (1971), however, equating play in early childhood with imaginative development. Arieti (1976) later explored creativity from a lifetime perspective of complex, mental, and analytical skills.

Defining "creativity" is difficult. There's a lack of agreement on what it is and how to measure it. And, studies on the creativity of older people are scarce. Some argue that a person becomes more flexible and adaptable as they age (Csikszentmihalyi, 1996; Komulainen, 1985; Reigel, 1973; Sasser-Coen, 1993). While these shifts may lead to a misinterpretation of a decline in cognitive and creative capacity, Sasser-Coen (1993) notes how creative changes can be attributed to cognitive changes as a result of cumulative living. Recent research has found that creative functions, and more specifically divergent thinking abilities, are preserved in older adulthood (Addis et al., 2016; Leon et al., 2014; Madore et al., 2016; Palmiero et al., 2014). Adnan et al. (2019) assert that divergent thinking associated with creativity expands with increased integration of functional brain networks.

Cognitive development continues to evolve throughout the lifespan. In late life, a person's thinking becomes more adaptable and flexible, a result of cognitive changes connected with long life experience. As the underlying thinking process evolves with age, a person's creative process and artistic style also evolve.

Cohen (2005) identified four attributes of the older brain that support the notion that through lived experience we develop a repertoire of strategies of adapting and coping: "The brain is continually resculpting itself in response to experience and learning; new brain cells *do* form throughout life; the brain's emotional circuitry matures and becomes more balanced with age; and the brain's two hemispheres are more equally used by older adults" (pp. 3–4). This means that the human brain continually improves upon its ability to understand complex human behavior. The older brain is more bilaterally integrated than younger brains for functions such as face recognition, working memory, and word retrieval. Bilateral brain adaptation is explored in more depth in chapter 8.

As the intrinsic thought process and personality changes with age and creative activity changes, the individual moves from culture-bound adherence to deeper self-reflection (Arnheim, 1986; Komulainen, 1985). Creativity's form and content vary with age. Youthful imagination is more spontaneous and intense (Arieti, 1976), whereas older artists create with greater purpose and introspection (Lubart & Sternberg, 1998).

Lubart and Sternberg's (1998) "Investment Theory" outlines the factors that contribute to changes in creativity of older people, including their enhanced ability to define and solve problems. The elder artist has a broader knowledge base to draw inspiration from. According to Lubart and Sternberg, the artist's intellectual style and personality also serve as sources of creativity.

Sinnot (1993) notes imagination shifts with maturity in parallel with post-formal thinking refinement. Because of this cognition and development growth, the older person has acquired the ability to engage creatively in various ways.

This concept emphasizes the creative process over the product. Instead of assessing the content of the artwork, Sinnot argues that increased creative thinking is present in the manner in which an older adult communicates with friends, family, and communities, as well as engaging in more traditional forms of creativity such as making art.

As noted, studies have shown that a person's thinking changes during aging, becoming more adaptable and flexible, and thus the creative process evolves. As a result, the individual becomes more introspective, more focused on an integrated work of art in which all elements of the composition are equal. This is in contrast to the work of younger artists for whom one element, such as an object with a strong light source, or a centralized, emphasized figure of power, overpowers the others. The self-portraits of Rembrandt van Rijn exemplify this theory, in which the paintings of his younger self appear in motion and with dynamic light contrast as compared with his self-portraits 30 and 50 years later in which he depicts himself seated and calmly facing forward, with subdued lighting across the fore and background.

Arnheim (1986) noted that, with age, the subject matter of artists' work tended to become more personal and introspective (e.g., Adeena's review of her life and Marcia's greater acceptance of death through more grounded spiritual beliefs). However, while Arnheim asserted that the work of older artists becomes more diffuse and generalized in composition and style, the artwork of these women did not appear to bear this out. In fact, their work appeared bolder and less homogenized.

Cohen-Shalev (1989) postulates that it may not be possible to generalize an old age style, especially across multiple media. In the mixed media and multi-dimensional work of Adeena, there is a a different set of aesthetic components than Marcia's two-dimensional acrylic paintings. Comparing their work and others in terms of an "old age style" is problematic. However, understanding a shift in style may help the artist to better understand her own work and process. A shift in style might also indicate a change in cognitive, emotional, or physical abilities, such as the case with Rose, who experienced more discomfort in holding and manipulating a pencil or brush. Noticing a shift may assist an art therapist or teaching artist in providing assistance or adaptive tools such as more light, or a longer or wider brush or pencil.

Influence of Art and Aging for Rose, Adeena, and Marcia

Cohen (2000) wrote about the importance for people at all ages to engage in a variety of creative activities. A range of creative endeavors, he proposed, not only gives us a palette from which to choose, but also an option should our health or abilities change. Some of these are more physically demanding, such as dancing and performing, while others are more sedentary, such as reading or drawing. Rose, Adeena, and Marcia were acutely aware of the benefit of creative activities and their impact on their lives.

These women did not speak about whether or not they felt they had become more or less creative with age, a topic upon which much of the literature is focused (Alpaugh et al., 1983; Dennis, 1966; Lehman, 1953; Sasser-Coen, 1993; Simonton, 1990), but being creative has been a persistent, lifelong attribute. This aligns with Kaufman's (2016) observation that creative identity is not a product of age but rather an ongoing self-perception established earlier in life.

This is consistent with the experience described by the artist Anne Truitt, who wrote about her life each day for one year (Truitt, 1982). She noted that although her artistic identity was rooted in childhood, it wasn't until she was in her 50s that she acknowledged herself as an artist.

Rather than being considered artists by others, what seemed to be most important to Rose, Adeena, and Marcia is that they considered themselves to be artists – that they felt it and believed it.

Researchers have stated that it is also important for aging women to have empathic relationships (Surrey, 1993) and to be connected with family and community (Browne, 1998). The experiences of Rose, Adeena, and Marcia support the literature contending that social connection is a vital component to feelings of satisfaction (Avlund et al., 1998; Bennett, 2002; Cohen et al., 2006; Fisher & Specht, 1999; Glass et al., 1999; Wikström, 2002). Social interaction and the creative process further contribute to personal growth, increased self-esteem, and an increased sense of purpose.

Leaving a Legacy

The literature that explores leaving a legacy in artwork (Magniant 2004; Spaniol, 1997) often focuses on how it is naturally tied to the life review, a natural process that occurs near the end of life. While this may be true, for these women leaving a legacy may have more to do with the developmental notions of Erikson (1959) and Tornstam (2005), according to which the aging individual feels compelled to share their knowledge with younger generations. The motivation to pass on ideas and stories also seems to be tied with notions of self-esteem and self-worth, particularly for Rose and Adeena, who felt that they had something important to say and that it should be shared.

Stanford (2006) found that women who had endured hardship early in life were better able to thrive in old age. Adeena's early life enduring WWII contributed to her strength, well-being, and self-esteem and served as a direct source of inspiration for her process of collecting and transforming materials. She also felt that her traumatic experience gave her tools to understand and express, artistically, the trauma of others. Rose's early family experience, in which she felt that she was always being put down and she wasn't good at anything, seems to have made her wiser and more self-aware. She became motivated to tell others how they, too, might believe in themselves. For all three of these women, passing knowledge and experience on to younger people was especially important.

In the interviews, much was discussed about changes in creative thinking, motivation, and identity. Each of these women expressed a greater need for self-expression as they grew older, and some of them felt more creative with age. As mentioned (Reed, 2005; Simonton, 1990), older adults have an increased capacity for creativity through the mastery and integration of life experiences. Sternberg and Lubart's (1993) perspective that a person's resources for creativity expand with life experience was apparent with all three women, who were increasingly able to draw from their life experiences, and some aging with a heightened level of motivation, like Adeena, who felt that her work was urgent, and Rose who was compelled to share her insight with others.

These three women's stories support the notion that a person's thinking becomes more flexible and adaptable with age (Cohen, 2005; Csikszentmihalyi, 1996; Sasser-Coen, 1993), and they themselves felt in many ways more creative as older women than before.

Their experience also supports the idea that as we age, we move from social conformity to introspection (Arnheim, 1986; Komulainen, 1985). Adeena expressed this in the way she dressed, the arrangement of her apartment, her artwork, and her method of trying to sell and exhibit it. Rose defied conformity in the way she taught art appreciation, inviting her students to look inward and find their own opinions and voice. Likewise, Marcia rejected conformity in not committing to explaining the meaning of her work. Rather, she was concerned with how the work looked and felt to her. She no longer cared about input or response from others.

Freedom to Experiment

Adeena, in particular, found that she had become more experimental in her work, in support of findings by Lindauer et al. (1997) that older artists had greater spontaneity and used abstraction more often, among other things. Lindauer et al. studied older professional artists and found that as they grew older, they reported an improvement in the quality and quantity of their artwork. The artists noted that they had learned more about themselves and their work, became more self-accepting and self-knowing, and became more active in local and global events. The artists attributed improvements to maturity and inspiration. Others reported more self-satisfaction. They were less concerned with criticism by others and felt more comfortable expressing themselves. The study showed significant differences between younger and older artists. Older artists thought they had special knowledge, including art training, life experience, and wisdom. More than half of artists felt their work was affected by physical and sensory changes, with some adjusting their techniques to work around physical limitations.

Rose, Adeena, and Marcia agreed that they became more creative as they aged and also felt a higher level of satisfaction in their work, a phenomenon noted by Lindauer, Orwoll, and Kelley in their 1997 study. Each of the three women mentioned that they grew less concerned about the opinions of others. They felt more comfortable in who they were and in expressing themselves. Rose and Adeena gained a greater understanding of themselves, which was expressed in their work. Adeena also attributed her growth to having more time as well as more confidence in her ability as she aged.

Physical Changes

Each of the women mentioned the loss or change of physical capabilities and its impact on their lives. However, these changes seemed to be outweighed by positive age-related emotional changes such as wisdom, motivation, and self-esteem closely related to their art-making.

Marcia had been severely limited by chronic fatigue syndrome just prior to the commencement of our interviews. Her poor physical health slowed down her creative process and limited her ability to leave home. But Marcia denied that her illness had any significant effect on the artwork itself. Instead, she insisted that art-making gave her motivation to get up and get to work every day, despite extreme fatigue. Her response might have been a result of her lifelong commitment to making art (Atchley, 1999), some level of transcendence over her physical limitations (Tornstam, 2005), or perhaps both.

Rose reported that arthritis affected the way she moved the brush and a decline in vision restricted her as well. She had been burdened by several illnesses and doctors' visits since our interviews began, and as a result, she was not able to work at her art or attend the open studio regularly. Rose, too, denied that the physical changes had a significant impact on her artwork, even though her physical limitations restricted her ability to go to museums and galleries, which had been an important component in her creative process.

Adeena did not report any particular physical changes or loss but rather spoke about the body getting old in a more general way. Mostly, she was concerned with time running out. At times, she mentioned physical ailments but did not indicate that this was a hindrance or detriment to her work.

Rose, Adeena, and Marcia each endured, to varying degrees, illness, injury, and physical changes due to aging, which had the potential to interfere with creative activities. Yet, each of them continued their involvement in art-making and other activities. Each acknowledged compensating for these age-related circumstances, but none said it was a major factor in how or why they make art; they accepted the physical changes and continued to work. It seemed that with regard to making art and the creative process, the impact of the emotional changes that arose with age seemed to outweigh the physical ones.

Conclusion

The ideas presented in this chapter are some ways to theoretically frame the work of art therapy with older people and creative aging, but they are in no way inclusive. My work with Rose, Adeena, and Marcia helped me understand what was important to each woman as she aged, in particular her creative outlook, creative processes, and how developing an identity as an artist can assist in reaching developmental benchmarks and confronting the challenges of aging.

Rose, Adeena, and Marcia generously shared with me their lives and what was important to them. From their stories and those of others with whom I've had the great fortune to work, I have formulated overarching goals that honor growth, wisdom, and self-actualization in old age by nurturing a sense of artistic identity; encouraging connection to oneself; and fostering a sense of purposefulness and motivation. These goals will be discussed in more detail in chapter 6.

References

Addis, D. R., Pan, L., Musicaro, R., & Schacter, D. L. (2016). Divergent thinking and constructing episodic simulations. *Memory*, *24*, 89–97. https://doi.org/10.1080/09658211.2014.985591

Adnan, A., Beaty, R., Silvia, P., Spreng, R. N., & Turner, G. R. (2019). Creative aging: Functional brain networks associated with divergent thinking in older and younger adults. *Neurobiology of Aging*, *75*, 150–158. https://doi.org/10.1016/j.neurobiolaging.2018.11.004

Alpaugh, P. K., Parham, I. A., Cole, K. D., & Birren, J. E. (1983). Creativity in adulthood and old age. *Educational Gerontology*, *1*, 17–40.

Arieti, S. (1976). *The intrapsychic self: Feeling, cognition, creativity in health and mental illness*. New York: Basic Books, Inc.

Arnheim, R. (1986). On the late style. In R. Arnheim (Ed.), *New essays on the psychology of art* (pp. 285–293). Berkeley, CA: University of California Press.

Atchley, R. C. (1999). *Continuity and adaptation in aging: Creating positive experiences*. Baltimore, MD: Johns Hopkins University Press.

Avlund, K, Damsgaard, M. T., & Holsten, B. E. (1998). Social relations and morality: An eleven year follow-up study of 70-yr-old men and women in Denmark. *Social Science & Medicine, 47*(5), 635–643.

Baltes, P. B., Smith, J., & Staudinger, U. M. (1992). Wisdom and successful aging. In T. Sonderegger (Ed.), *Nebraska symposium on motivation* (pp. 123–167). Lincoln, NE: University of Nebraska Press.

Bennett, K. M. (2002). Low level social engagement as a precursor of mortality among people in later life. *Age and Ageing, 31*, 165–168.

Browne, C. V. (1998). *Women, feminism and aging.* New York: Springer.

Butler, R. N. (1963). The life review: An interpretation of reminiscence in the aged. *Psychiatry, 26*, 65–76.

Cohen, G. D. (2000). *The Creative Age: Awakening human potential in the second half of life.* New York: Avon Books/Harper Collins Publishers.

Cohen, G. D. (2005). *The mature mind: The positive power of the aging brain.* New York: Basic Books.

Cohen, G. D., Perlstein, S., Chapline, J., Kelly, J., Firth, K. M., & Simmens, S. (2006). The impact of professionally conducted cultural programs on the physical health, mental health, and social functioning of older adults. *The Gerontologist, 46*(6), 726–734.

Cohen-Shalev, A. (1989). Old age style: Developmental changes in creative production from a life-span perspective. *Journal of Aging Studies, 3*(1), 21–37.

Csikszentmihalyi, M. (1996). *Creativity: Flow and the psychology of discovery and invention.* New York: HarperCollins Publishers, Inc.

Dennis, W. (1966). Creative productivity between the ages of 20 and 80 years. *Journal of Gerontology, 21*, 1–8.

Diehl, M., & Wahl, H.-W. (2020). Risks and potentials of adult development and aging: Understanding the challenges and opportunities of successful aging. In *The psychology of later life: A contextual perspective* (pp. 153–180). American Psychological Association. https://doi-org.ezproxyles.flo.org/10.1037/0000185-007

Erikson, E. H. (1959) *Identity and the life cycle.* New York: Norton

Erikson, E. H., & Erikson, J. M. (1997). *The life cycle completed: Extended version with new chapters on the Ninth Stage of development.* New York: W.W. Norton & Company, Inc.

Fisher, B. J., & Specht, D. K. (1999). Successful aging and creativity in later life. *Journal of Aging Studies, 13*(4), 457–472.

Freud, S. (1952). *On dreams.* New York: W.W. Norton & Company, Inc.

Glass, T. A., de leon, C. M., Marottoli, R. A., & Berkman, L. F. (1999). Population-based study of social and productive activities as predictors of survival among elderly Americans. *British Medical Journal, 319*, 478–483.

Kaufman, J. C. (2016). *Creativity 101* (2nd ed.). Springer Publishing Company.

Komulainen, S. P. J. (1985). Creative abilities as a life-span phenomenon: A crosscut survey in Finland. *Creative Child and Adults Quarterly, 10*(3), 170–181.

Kris, E. (1952). *Psychoanalytic explorations in art.* International Universities Press.

Lehman, H. C. (1953). *Age and achievement.* Princeton, NJ: Princeton University Press/American Philosophical Society.

Leon, S. A., Altmann, L. J. P., Abrams, L., Gonzalez, R. L. J., & Heilman, K. M. (2014). Divergent task performance in older adults: Declarative memory or creative potential? *Creativity Research Journal, 26*, 21–29. https://doi.org/10.1080/10400419.2014.873657

Lindauer, M. S., Orwoll, L., & Kelley, M. C. (1997). Aging artists on the creativity of their old age. *Creativity Research Journal, 10*(2–3), 133–152.

Lubart, T. I., & Sternberg, R. J. (1998). Life span creativity: An investment theory approach. In C. E. Adams-Price (Ed.), *Creativity and successful aging: Theoretical and empirical approaches* (pp. 21–41). New York: Springer Publishing Company.

Madore, K. P., Jing, H. G., & Schacter, D. L. (2016). Divergent creative thinking in young and older adults: Extending the effects of an episodic specificity induction. *Memory & Cognition, 44*, 974e988.

Magniant, R. C. P. (2004). *Art therapy with older adults: A sourcebook.* Springfield, IL: Charles C. Thomas Publisher, Ltd.

Maslow, A. (1968). *Towards a psychology of being* (2nd ed.). New York: Van Nostrand Reinhold Company Inc.

Palmiero, M., Giacomo, D. D., & Passafiume, D. (2014). Divergent thinking and age-related changes. *Creativity Research Journal, 26*, 456–460. https://doi.org/10.1080/10400419.2014.961786

Rank, O. (1932). *Art and artist: Creative urge and personality development.* New York: W.W. Norton.

Reed, I. (2005). Creativity: Self-perceptions over time. *International Journal of Aging and Human Development, 60*(1), 1–18.

Reigel, K. F. (1973). Dialectical operations: The final period of cognitive development. *Human Development, 16*, 346–370.

Sasser-Coen, J. R. (1993). Qualitative changes in creativity in the second half of life: A life-span developmental perspective. *Journal of Creative Behavior, 27*(1), 18–27.

Simonton, D. K. (1990). Does creativity decline in the later years? In M. Perlmutter (Ed.), *Late life potential* (pp. 83–112). Washington, DC: The Gerontological Society of America.

Sinnot, J. D. (1993). Creativity and postformal thought: Why the last stage is the creative stage. In C. E. Adams-Price, (Ed.), *Creativity and successful aging: Theoretical and empirical approaches* (pp. 43–72). New York: Springer.

Spaniol, S. (1997). Art therapy with older adults: Challenging myths, building competencies. *Art Therapy, 14*(3), 158–160.

Stanford, B. H. (2006). Through wise eyes: Thriving elder women's perspective on thriving in elder adulthood. *Educational Gerontology, 32*(10), 881–905.

Sternberg, Robert J., & Lubart, Todd I. (1993). Investing in creativity. *Psychological Inquiry, 4*(3), 229–232. doi:10.1207/s15327965pli0403_16

Stowe, J. D., & Cooney, T. M. (2015). Examining Rowe and Kahn's concept of successful aging: Importance of taking a life course perspective. *Gerontologist, 55*(1), 43–50. doi:10.1093/geront/gnu055

Surrey, J. L. (1993). Self-in-relations: A theory of women's development. *Advanced Development, 5*, 1–11.

Tornstam, L. (2005). *Gerotranscendence: A developmental theory of positive aging.* New York: Springer Publishing Company.

Truitt, A. (1982). Daybook. New York: Pantheon Books.

Wikström, B. M. (2002). Social interaction associated with visual art discussions: A controlled intervention study. *Aging & Mental Health, 6*(1), 82–87.

Winnicott, D. W. (1971). *Playing and reality.* London: Tavistock Publications.

4 Back in My Day

"I feel that everybody is worth remembering..." – Adeena

The arts have the potential to serve as a powerful intergenerational bridge spanning historical and sociocultural differences. Recognizing and responding to the influence of these differences contributes to heightened sensitivity and a broader understanding of human development across generations. In arts programs, this gives rise to a greater appreciation of the program participants and, perhaps most important, to culturally competent therapeutic encounters, in which there is awareness of the differences in history, culture, and aesthetic between the therapist and the participant, and between participants themselves.

Developing Intergenerational Understanding

The historical moment in which a generation lives impacts a wide range of cultural beliefs not always shared by subsequent generations. In an arts program, in particular, intergenerational work is about bringing generations together, but it is also about the relationship between the younger therapist or teaching artist and the participants. Social development needs to be considered in the context of the respective cohort's socialization – or, in other words, their unique social experiences and motivations.

Bühler and Nikitin (2020) note, for example, how many theories of adult development are based on cohorts who were born in the first half of the last century, reaching young adulthood during the Great Depression, World War II, and the postwar era. These historical events defined the course of their lives, affected their career options, and influenced their decisions to prioritize family. Adults born in the second half of the last century were socialized by a different set of historical episodes, setting them on a different life course, with its own opportunities and priorities. Anachronistic or culturally conditioned lifespan development models must be replaced by ones that reflect the modern era.

I experienced a deeply reflective moment while teaching a course on creativity and aging to a class of art therapy students in Estonia. It was a moment that made me see how my perspective is based upon my own history and culture. I was telling the students about Maslow's hierarchy of needs when their eyes glazed over. I stopped and asked, "Whoah! What just happened? I just lost you ..." The students replied that the theory didn't feel right when thinking about the older generation in Estonia. They explained that many people in the older generation were still in need of, or felt at risk of losing, basic needs such as food and shelter, and so the idea of "self-actualization," the top rung of Maslow's signature-needs pyramid, was not relevant. Since then, I have been reflecting on how American history and culture, as well as my own personal history and culture, have informed my work and research. It has made me think about the assumptions I make. Now I recognize how important it is to examine my premises and assumptions, both for myself and for the art therapists who work intergenerationally.

I later returned to Estonia to implement a new creative arts therapy program for older adults and to train the students and clinicians who worked there. During that visit, two other moments left an impression on me.

In one of the nursing homes, the younger students and staff spoke Estonian, but the older residents spoke only Russian. The language disparity was directly linked to the Soviet Occupation of Estonia from 1944 to 1991, in which Russian replaced the Estonian language for many people. Since Estonia regained independence, only Estonian and English are taught to students thus most of the interns spoke those languages. Despite these language differences, students and staff reported that the visual language of art allowed them to communicate. Setting out art materials and visual tools such as photographs of art and architecture allowed the older adults and clinicians to play, collaborate, and develop relationships.

At the same nursing home, one of the therapists told me that an older gentleman with dementia who had just moved in was having a particularly difficult time. While adjustment difficulties are not uncommon for people with dementia when they are uprooted from their homes and moved to an unfamiliar place, it was particularly acute for this man, who thought he had been sent to a gulag in Siberia. It is possible that he had actually spent time in a gulag during the Soviet era, or perhaps the threat of being sent to one had loomed large throughout much of his life. That moving to a nursing home could reignite this kind of trauma in an already frail individual was startling. It made me wonder if something could have been done differently in his transition to prevent this frightening and confusing experience. For example, would knowing more about his family history have helped the nursing home staff communicate with him differently? Are there ways to identify such a risk ahead of time?

I remembered David, a kind man with Alzheimer's disease who had recently moved from his home onto the dementia-care floor of an assisted living facility. He was confused and depressed, desperate to go home. He thought that his family had abandoned him. His wife reported that since his move, his recall of the names of his family members had worsened. I had the opportunity to work with him in a few individual art therapy sessions. An architect, his drawing skills were exceptional.

In my presence, he worked on a cityscape drawing using fine-tip, high-quality architectural pens, which I surmised were tools very familiar to him. The perspective of this large, complicated drawing of very tall buildings in an urban landscape was from ground level, with skyscrapers leaning darkly overhead, unmoored and tilting inward. The drawing evoked for me a sense of being trapped, frightened, and out of control. At the same time, it was drawn with a high level of skill that evoked confident intentionality about the imagery and its execution. His wife then showed me a collection of his earlier paintings that were more typical of his work. These works were also highly skilled but far more technically refined. More realistic, they included utilization of a full-color palette and naturalistic perspective. Without seeing David's former artwork, I would not have grasped just how lost he was feeling. I did not have the opportunity to work with him beyond our few sessions, but his art made clear his difficulty adjusting to the assisted living residence, and was the occasion for subsequent conversations between his wife, me, and the assisted living staff aimed at bolstering the support he needed to make the transition more comfortable.

A Framework of Intergenerational Inquiry

Drawing from my personal experiences as an art therapist and art therapy educator and my experiences working and teaching abroad, it makes sense to me to frame intergenerational inquiry using three categories: historical, cultural, and aesthetic. These categories include, respectively, the historical context that impacted a specific generation – their arts, language, and traditions, and finally, their tastes, such as visual and musical preferences. Alongside the backdrop of generational/cohort-wide influences, family and person-specific history, culture, and aesthetic influences must also be considered.

By recognizing the historical and cultural moments in which I, as well as my clients, grew up and live, I am able to take steps to understand the societal environment that shapes our lives. Of course, an older person will see the world differently than I do. My intention is that in learning about that vantage point in comparison with my own, I can break apart ageist assumptions and replace them with meaningful relationships with individuals of a different generation.

Historical Context

The experiences I had in Estonia, in particular, helped me to see how the history of each generation, cohort, and individual has a formative impact. While I understood this on one level, having worked with older adults for many years, I was blind to some of these issues in my own country. Many of the people I worked with had lived through the Great Depression and WWII or had fled Europe and resettled in New York, where I was living. But, working with relatively privileged people, I didn't really understand what it meant to be hungry, or to be a child fleeing war. I did not understand the impact events like these had on the rest of one's life, how one is forever changed by such experiences, and how they create a lens through which everything that follows is viewed.

Across many countries worldwide, for people born roughly between 1920 and 1940, the impact of World War II looms large. The vast devastation, genocide, and migrations of that war make it in many respects the singular most impactful historical event of the older generation. Its impact is felt broadly and acutely, from the societal structures that ruptured and regrew, reframing how life was lived, to the more personal impact of war on a family, such as the death of a soldier or destruction of home or livelihood. The younger postwar generations in the United States, on the other hand, have had relative peace and social and economic opportunity. How does a person from the younger generation understand the experience of those who came of age before the war?

A young Jewish child living with her family in London during World War II, Adeena was sent to the countryside with thousands of other children for protection from the Blitz bombing in London. From there she was treated for tuburculosis at a medical facility, where she remained until the end of the war, recuperating. Her disease was horribly debilitating at the time, which, along with the separation from her family and fear of the war, had a lasting impact on the young adolescent. Her early life enduring WWII contributed to her strength, well-being, and self-esteem and have served as a source of inspiration for her artwork. She felt pressed to share the story – to pass along the history – but also in her process of collecting and transforming materials. She explained, "I feel a sense of urgency to make art because I want people to know what happened to me. I feel I am a representative of the Jews, of the Holocaust. I feel I have a great deal to offer in terms of history ..." She also feels that her traumatic experience gives her tools to understand and express, artistically, the trauma of others.

Moving into a new apartment – and perhaps also the closeness of death, as many of her neighbors are elderly – triggered Adeena's war experiences of dislocation. She explained:

> My thoughts about my childhood and the Holocaust have something to do with age. I mean, I've read about why these things often do

come out when you're older. There are two reasons I can think of. One is that you're confronting the hugest loss because I certainly think about death now. I never did before. How is it coming? When is it coming?

I wonder, is Adeena at risk of being retraumatized, like the Estonian man who thought he had been sent to a gulag when he was relocated to a nursing home?

Culture

I define "culture" as the customs, shared beliefs and attitudes, values, goals, and practices of a particular group of people. It is difficult to look at culture from a wide-angle lens. There are so many variations of beliefs, customs, and arts. How much is culture changed by historical moments, and how is cultural identity retained through periods of oppression? The arts are a powerful tool for coping with the stress and trauma associated with these large historical moments, but it is perhaps more critical to look on a micro level at the culture of the group or groups to which an older adult as well as their caregiver belong than it is to look at the macro level of the historical moment.

One cross-nation cultural comparison relevant to this book is the social support and infrastructure available for the care of older adults. In the United States, there are many established social and care services available to older adults and their families. In lieu of caring for family members at home, many take advantage of these services. In some cases, they are utilized to help an older person live independently longer. There are also special care facilities for older people with dementia, such as Alzheimer's disease. By comparison, the social services available to older adults in Estonia exist primarily in more urban areas; in Ukraine, I learned from Ukrainian art therapists and psychologists, they barely exist at all. There are, of course, socioeconomic reasons behind the discrepancies, but the tradition for elders to remain in the home in the absence of resources such as nursing homes, and ageist attitudes about older adults' value in society play a role. These respective patterns affect the degree of creative arts therapy available to older adults.

Another cultural impact on creative arts therapy is the overall role of the arts in society. The visual and performing arts in the United States often hold an elite position in society. Housed in marbled museums and gilded theaters, access to them is out of reach for many. In light of such variations in access to culture, I have tried to understand what is thought of as "art" in a particular country or region. Where are the arts situated? Given their status or lack thereof, how can they best be accessed in our work? And what is the generational experience of this? For example, what is it like for an older person in a place like Estonia or Ukraine, where arts had once flourished, then were suppressed during Soviet occupation, to see the younger generations resurrecting traditional arts? How can these traditional arts be used intergenerationally? While teaching in Estonia, I learned that my students' training in the arts was different than that of my American students. While my American students were trained in painting, sculpture, and photography, many of my Estonian students were trained in handicrafts like fiber arts and ceramics. Also, I learned that in Estonia singing is the most important art form, revered for carrying forth centuries-old Estonian traditions.

Paul was a lively man with Alzheimer's disease. He was eager to participate in some of the activities in the dementia day program and resistant to others. He was especially resistant to engage in art-making when I first began with him. He had been the lead actor in the dementia day program's production of *My Fair Lady*, so I knew that he enjoyed being part of the program activities and had the capacity for creative expression. His resistance seemed to stem from the fact that I was a stranger to him and that he was unfamiliar with visual art-making. I needed to go slowly to build a relationship with him while at the same time modeling how visual expression works, using a variety of art media in his presence. Paul frequently talked about the New York Yankees. Enthused by the topic of baseball, at every turn he was eager to share his opinion about various players, although most of them had played long ago.

One day, the "all-time All-Star New York Yankees team" was the topic of conversation. Taking the opportunity to connect with him on something he cared about that was deeply rooted in his identity as a New Yorker, I asked him details about which player was the All-Star for various positions – pitcher, catcher, first baseman, and so on. Methodically, we listed, by position, the best Yankees players of all time. From there, I cut baseball players from construction paper and a baseball diamond. Each player was named and then placed in their appropriate position on the diamond. The result was a visual display of Paul's *Yankees All-Time All-Star Team*, for which he was proud and delighted. This activity was an important bridge in my relationship with him, securing his trust by evidencing that I cared about him and was curious to know him. It also demonstrated to him how an idea can be expressed in a visual way. From then on, Paul was an eager participant in visual art activities and was prolific in independently creating artwork.

Aesthetics

I refer to aesthetics as the general tastes, preferences, and sensibility of a generation, expressed in the arts (visual, dance, drama, music), industrial and graphic design, architecture, speech, and language. Although aesthetic tastes are found at a more individualized level than culture, at the same time, they are shaped by the times we live in, and the aesthetic dimension is a powerful way to reflect the pulse of what is happening to a group at any given point in time. While I don't think it is possible to generalize about taste, a younger person in the United States is likely to have more tolerance for experiencing a multiplicity of images simultaneously, including quick-moving images on a screen or iPad, while an older person might feel overwhelmed by them.

Aesthetics influence my work as an art therapist, for they frame how my clients and I express ourselves visually. This plays out in a number of ways in my work with older people. Are the images I present congruent with my client's aesthetic tastes? Does my pacing of the session foster in them the flow of creativity and imagination? Is the background music I find soothing experienced as sensory overload for that person?

Joe worked as an industrial designer. His career, designing furniture and appliances, spanned roughly 40 years in the mid-20th century. Like David, whose livelihood relied on drawing, Joe's artwork, even as a 90-year-old with advanced Alzheimer's, continued to reflect the influence of mid-century design. One example of this was his painting *Mid-Century Sunflower* (Figure 4.1[1] Mid-Century Sunflower). While the shape and color resemble the sunflower, in particular the yellow outer rings and brown circle, the squared-off edges and simplification of a complex object reflects mid-century industrial design. Although Joe was unable to tell us about the aesthetic influences in his designs, his artwork spoke for him. Understanding Joe better was helpful in developing a richer relationship with him and allowed us to be more thoughtful and purposeful in our approach to art-making with him.

I describe these differences as a way to illustrate generational and intergenerational influences on the way in which we see life and express ourselves. It is difficult to understand the life experience of another, let alone grasp the historical and cultural factors that shaped them, especially when they came up a generation before or after we did. But, doing our best to know ourselves very well and learning the best we can about those we are serving is vital.

Exploratory Questions

In an effort to encourage my art therapy students to explore their own identity, I introduce an art-making experiential in which they are asked to make a visual representation of the following question: What are some of the historical, cultural, and aesthetic influences on your life? Next, students share this visual representation and their realizations about it with a classmate, discussing the following questions: How are your experiences similar/different to those of your client(s) (or peers, or colleagues)? How have these experiences shaped your identity as an art therapist?

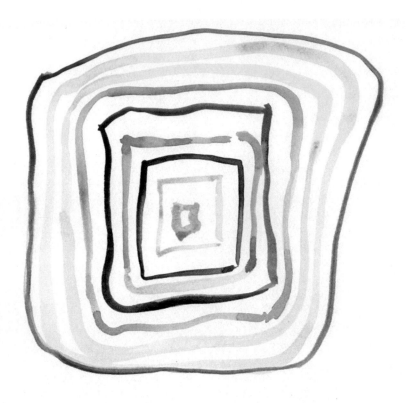

Figure 4.1 Mid-Century Sunflower.

I have given this experiential to students and arts in health practitioners in the United States, Ukraine, and Estonia. After facilitating this experiential via Skype to a group of ten Ukrainian art therapists in Lviv, I also offered it to my students at Lesley University. As you might expect, they expressed strikingly different influences. Many variables besides their lived experience may have been influential – e.g., face-to-face vs. online interaction, direct communication vs. my need for a translator, the younger age of the American students vs. the slightly older ages of the Ukrainian audience, not to mention my own role of authority as professor of a semester-long graded course vs. an hour-long guest lecturer from far away via computer.

The Ukrainian art therapists spent most of their time speaking about historical influences. While the American students noted a few historical events, most often 9/11, they focused largely on cultural influences, teasing out what they meant for each person. At the time, the conflict with Russia in Eastern Ukraine was heated. Several Ukrainian art therapists linked the Chernobyl nuclear disaster to the current conflict. I was curious about how they connected these events, which occurred 30 years apart. Culture and aesthetics were not discussed among the Ukrainian art therapists, but they were eager to tell me about generational trauma.

While the American art therapy students were far more invested in exploring cultural influences, "culture" for these students was associated with the culture and ethnicity of their families of origin, and for each of them, that was uniquely different. I wondered, was culture a more influential concept for this generation of students than history was for the Ukrainian art therapists? Was the exploration of culture more pronounced with this group because it is frequently discussed among the student cohort and in the training program? My limited observations were in no way a formal study, and the point of the exercise was in any case for the participants and students themselves to become curious about their lives and those with whom they were working. However, curiosity about the responses of each cohort might lead to further exploration and a deeper understanding of the lived experience of these participants, of how their experience differs from my own, and how I can bridge difference to become a more empathic, culturally competent therapist or teacher.

Exploring the history, culture, and aesthetics of those with whom we work, I seek to understand the intergenerational implications of history, culture, and aesthetics in my work as an art therapist and creative arts therapy educator. The Covid-19 pandemic, during which I am writing this book, will surely be another impactful historical – and cultural – event that will shape each generation alive at this time, and in different ways.

The following points, drawn from a broader gerontological and sociological perspective, are also worth considering with regard to arts therapy and creative aging:

- What are the implications of the socioeconomic situation of each generation?
- What are their attitudes about giving or receiving care outside the family unit?
- How does (political and economic) history influence social services? And how do they influence society's attitudes toward aging?
- How has immigration shaped the comparative views and experiences of generations?
- How has intergenerational trauma manifested itself? How does this play out between older adult and caregiver?
- What can we learn from exploring other nations, regions, and cultures? Does it help our students to examine their own?

It is not enough to simply care about the people we work with. We must do our best to understand where they are coming from and what their lived experience has been.

Note

1 This image has been redrawn by the author due to poor photographic quality of the original work.

Reference

Bühler, J. L., & Nikitin, J. (2020). Sociohistorical context and adult social development: New directions for 21st century research. *American Psychologist*, *75*(4), 457–469.

5   Intersections of Care

This chapter begins a more directed look into how the arts can be applied in the care of older adults. The previous chapters offered a platform of how arts are beneficial for the health and well-being of older people. This and the following chapters detail the practice of art therapy and creative aging.

As an art therapist who presents to audiences beyond my immediate field, I am often asked about the difference between art therapy and creative aging, especially with the emergence of creative aging practices, in which professional artists are employed to share their artistic practice with older people. The wider field of creative aging encompasses art therapists, teaching artists, and others who harness the arts in a wide range of ways for the benefit of health. This not only provides direct benefit to the older person but also utilizes art to improve environments in which health care takes place.

Art therapists are trained in a practice that integrates psychology and art and involves extensive clinical training and preparation for accreditation and licensing. In some circumstances, an art therapist is the most appropriate choice for providing care; in others, a teaching artist – a professional in their artistic craft – is a better choice. In many cases, in working with older people, either is a good choice. So much of this work is grounded in empathy, resting on a caregiver's ability to put themselves in the position of another, to understand their situation and point of view. The core of the work is relational, developing a connection with another and using that relationship (and with it, the art-making) for the benefit of the client. That means that the caregiver adapts to the needs of the cared for. Through empathic understanding, the caregiver can understand what that person needs, the barriers to meeting that need, and the best form of therapeutic work to bridge those barriers.

Practitioners of art therapy and creative aging each have unique assets and training, and yet there is overlap among them. Rather than playing a turf war, I prefer to view both these groups of arts professionals as well-positioned to improve the health and well-being of older people. With an ever-growing population of older people in our society, surely the need

Table 5.1 Venn Diagram of Creative Aging and Art Therapy

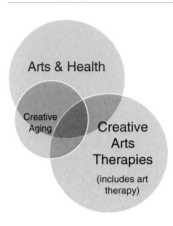

for arts programs far outweighs our differences over who can provide them. Nobody owns the arts, and yet all of us can benefit.

Creative art therapists and creative aging practitioners all believe that engagement in the arts can help alleviate suffering, whether it be mental, physical, social, or spiritual. What, then, are the distinctions between them? Referring to the Venn diagram (Table 5.1), this chapter will identify the distinct characteristics of each as well as their overlapping commonalities.

This discussion is in no way definitive, but rather is an attempt to sort out when and why an art therapist might be better suited than a creative aging teaching artist, and vice versa. It will also explore the vast opportunity for all therapists and artists who specialize in working with older people to meet a huge need.

Art Therapy

Art therapy is an integrative mental health and human services profession, helping people cope with mental health problems as well as those seeking emotional, creative, and spiritual growth. Art therapy has traditionally been known as a psychotherapy approach that uses visual art as a springboard to gain deeper insight. Early art therapists Margaret Naumburg (1950) and Edith Kramer (1971), among others, used psychoanalytic ideas in their practice, focusing on both the creative process and product. Subsequently, art therapy has evolved alongside the development of theories of psychology, such as gestalt, cognitive-behavioral, humanistic, and critical theory. Contemporary art therapy practice, while still rooted in psychotherapy, is increasingly practiced to support and lift marginalized communities (Timm-Bottos, 2016).

Art therapy theories and techniques blend concepts of art and psychology as a means to deepen the human experience through visual expression. Art therapists have a deep understanding of human and creative development, broad theoretical knowledge stemming from psychology, and extensive supervised clinical training in the application of art therapy approaches and methods. They learn and practice a range of formal and informal assessments and are equipped to assess mood, possible illness, and artistic interest and ability, and more. With honed skills in treatment planning, art therapists develop and implement interventions and experiences tailored to the specific cognitive, emotional, social, and physical needs of the client. Art therapists acquire a 60-credit master's degree in art therapy, which includes substantial classroom and practical training; significant post-graduate supervised work is required to receive the Registered Art Therapist (ATR) credential, board certification (ATR-BC) and/or a state license in art therapy or mental health counseling. Art therapy education is accredited, and registration and state licensure are regulated.

The practice of art therapy with older people covers a wide spectrum. Art therapists work with mental illness, cognitive impairment, and physical loss or change, as well as with those who are simply seeking enrichment. They are trained to notice subtleties in behavior and in the artwork that provide a deeper understanding of a person. In session, art therapists discern shifts in artistic or emotional expression and are trained to make appropriate interventions where necessary. They are also often able to recognize the onset of illness such as dementia before other clinicians, as the illness may show up in the artwork or art-making before it is detectable elsewhere. For example, an art therapist can recognize nuances in a person's drawings, such as broken lines or a peculiar placement of objects in space that might indicate disorganization or early dementia.

Art therapists are employed across the spectrum of health care services and can make referrals if additional treatment is needed. For example, in geriatric psychiatry, art therapists work with a treatment team of psychiatrists, nurses, social workers, and sometimes occupational therapists and other professionals. This treatment milieu works to help to reduce or eliminate the symptoms of acute mental illness in the patients. They work in hospice to help people cope with death and dying and with people who have impaired verbal interaction stemming from dementia, stroke, aphasia, Parkinson's, and other causes. Art therapy can also be used to:

• Develop self-awareness and introspection
• Offer elders a chance to connect with peers and other generations
• Facilitate life review
• Leave family and friends a legacy
• Help older people broaden their interests and experiences

- Help them cope with physical limitations through the use of adaptive techniques and expressive tools
- Heal communities and individuals experiencing trauma

The Third Hand

The art therapist's "third hand" is especially useful when working with older adults with cognitive or physical limitations. Often a person cannot completely implement their creative ideas and needs the use of the versatility, ingenuity, or technical knowledge of the therapist. In her work with children, Kramer (1986) illustrated how the artistic abilities and imagination of the art therapist are used in the empathic execution of the client's creative intent. Naming this type of therapeutic aid the "third hand," Kramer described it not as a therapeutic intervention but as a client "extension." The third hand, she explained, is "a hand that helps the creative process along without being intrusive, without distorting meaning or imposing pictorial ideas or preferences alien to the client" (1986, p. 71).

In this way, the art therapist relies on their artistic ability to execute the client's artistic intentions; in the process, however, the therapist should try to mirror or impose the client's artistic style. It is therefore important that the therapist understand the client's level of cognitive and creative development as well as their psychic and functional needs, so that interventions can be implemented appropriately.

In working with older adults, when the individual has lost the ability to set up workspace and art materials, the art therapist can do so. The third hand can then be invoked to deal with dripping paint or steady a teetering sculpture, or act as an "auxiliary hand" for individuals with physical limitations, undertaking the actual execution of placing strokes of paint on the canvas or applying and moving bits of clay to a sculpture (Kramer, 1986). Henley (1995) also suggests that the art studio itself can essentially function as a third hand, as it provides the environment for self-expression and creative engagement. The concept of the third hand is a central concept in art therapy work and is useful both in understanding how art therapy is practiced and in explaining some of the goals of art programs for older adults offered in this book.

Creative Aging

Creative aging is a field related to but distinct from the creative arts therapies. Creative aging professionals incorporate the arts into a wide range of health institutions and community support services. Creative aging is often understood as a field existing under the umbrella of arts in health. The arts in health movement emerged in the 1980s and 1990s as a holistic alternative or adjunctive option to the medical model of care.

Recognized for its healing abilities, it has been cultivated across a broad range of health care practices and institutions.

Creative aging has evolved rapidly in the past decade in the United States. Creative aging includes a broad spectrum of art professionals working with older adults. This includes professional artists or "teaching artists," creative arts therapists, art educators, physicians, nurses, social workers, and health care administrators, to name a few, along with elders and their care partners participating in creative aging programs.

Creative aging professionals provide vital services for aging Americans, helping them live independently and improving health and well-being for those in assisted care. The creative aging movement has also helped change the public debate from a focus on disease and marginalization to a more favorable perception of elders' capacities, abilities, and potential. Increasingly, the goals of art therapy with older adults overlap with the expansion of our understanding of creativity and aging. The current creative aging methodology includes the teaching and practice of art and its utilization as a tool for life enhancement.

Hanna et al. (2015) outline the three main areas of creative aging – arts in health care, lifelong learning, and universal design. Creative aging care integrates arts interventions in clinical settings, where arts therapists and professional artists team with health care practitioners to deliver a holistic focus on a person's strengths and abilities, shifting from the medical model that sees aging as a time of loss of functioning. Lifelong learning and community engagement encourage active participation in the arts as vital to quality of life, economic vitality, and reduced health care costs (Cantu & Fleuriet, 2018; Cohen et al., 2007). Universal design underscores the importance of the livability of homes and communities that reflect resident choice. This includes extending the ability to age in place, thereby supporting autonomy and well-being, and reducing long-term care costs.

Creative aging practitioners have devoted their attention to their own art and thus bring a high level of artistry to their work. Often, they are themselves professional artists or "teaching artists," which can mean that they have done advanced study in fine art and are ongoing learners and practitioners of their craft. These professionals have a wealth of experience and a passion for their work, and many have received training in how to engage older people in art-making. The training criteria for creative aging professionals are not formalized, but some programs, such as the Arts for the Aging Teaching Artist Institute, include initial training workshops and ongoing learning (discussed later in this chapter). Creative aging practitioners are empathic people who have an attuned ability to manipulate art-making to serve the needs and abilities of those with whom they work. Unlike the creative arts therapies, there currently does not exist licensure or credentialing for creative aging professionals.

Trained to attune to individual signs of engagement, enjoyment, and the promotion of overall health and well-being, creative aging practitioners provide humanizing, creative experiences that are complementary to their clients' overall health goals. The practice of creative aging centers artistic expression as a way to foster self-esteem, confidence, happiness, and a sense of achievement. This method follows an approach quite different from the traditional art course or museum program in that the focus is on building relationships between participants and community, and in many ways aligns more with art therapy practice.

Creative aging might also be referred to as lifelong learning. Broad in its application, lifelong learning includes museum education programs, community-based learning, and programs in higher education. Museum programs designed for older people, including those with dementia and their care partners, have been successful and popular in museums across the world. The Museum of Modern Art (MoMA) in New York has been a leader in museum education. Their innovative programs make the museum collection accessible for visitors with a range of disabilities, including dementia. Similarly, Livingston et al. (2016) noted how art-looking and art-making in the Art in the Moment program at the Art Institute of Chicago supported participants and were self-affirming. A program evaluation by Bennington et al. (2016) of an art therapy program in an art museum that incorporated observation of art and art-making drew a similar conclusion – that participants' well-being and social connection increased.

Intersection of Art Therapy and Creative Aging

Each person has the capacity for creativity and imagination and therefore can express themselves through art. This fundamental belief is shared across these two fields. One of the greatest aspects of the human mind is its ability to use symbols and metaphors to communicate. Through creativity and imagination, we are able to invent new technologies, make music, paint something that has never ever been seen, and write stories that shock or soothe our soul. This underlying premise is the foundation for both art therapy and creative aging. Another shared belief is that the arts are healing and improve our life experience. Even without intervention from therapists or teaching artists, the arts can be healing; however, the adaptations employed by therapists and arts in health practitioners can tailor that accessibility to attain greater benefits. Art is all about taking risk; it offers a great opportunity for self-learning through introspection, attainment of new skills, and never-ending possibilities for creating something new.

Of course, goals are very much tailored to the participant, depending on that person's needs, abilities, and the nature of the arts experience.

However, the underlying goals of most art therapy and creative aging programs are similar and include the following:

- Drawing out the potential in each person
- Promoting imagination
- Building and celebrating community
- Overcoming and coping with challenges
- Promoting life enhancement and well-being
- Encouraging personal development
- Providing knowledge and skill-building where appropriate

Both art therapy and creative aging utilize person-centered practices that place the experience of the participants front and center, with the goal of empowering them. At the same time, both have a critical theory perspective that works to dismantle negative perceptions about aging and eradicate the marginalization of older people in our society. Here, the art-making process is more about cultivating awareness than creating an art object. Therefore, learning happens by exploring the experience of a person or group in a way that recognizes the participant as the expert. They have the voice and space to communicate their experiences.

Art therapists and creative aging practitioners are trained to identify the abilities and potential barriers of those with whom they work and can be effective partners for older adults at any stage or situation in life. Through the cultivation of relationships, the skilled practitioner is able to employ art-making for focused purposes that go beyond enjoyment to foster empowerment, insight, and mastery, along with a whole host of mental health benefits, such as improved mood, mobility, etc. Art therapists are highly trained in the purposeful employment of art to benefit health. The most important aspect of any art therapy and creative aging encounter is that it is adapted to the unique needs and abilities of its participants. Art therapists and teaching artists provide access to the arts through their ability to inspire and their teaching skills, by creating opportunities, adapting tools, and more. Practitioners in each field understand lifespan development and draw from this knowledge in developing programs and experiences appropriate to the developmental stages of older people.

Example of an Art Therapy Program

New York University Creative Aging Therapeutic Program

The New York University Creative Aging Therapeutic Services (NYU CATS) offered free-of-charge art therapy services to underserved older adults in New York City and provided supervised training for graduate art therapy students. Funded by a grant from the Werner Dannheisser Testamentary Trust, NYU CATS partnered with two pre-existing programs serving older adults in NYC. This partnership allowed them to focus funds and attention directly on service delivery rather than on logistics such as renting a space, utility costs, transportation, marketing, and personnel recruitment. One partnership was with the Lenox Hill Neighborhood House Center for of Alzheimer's Respite (CARE) Program, a social adult day for people with advanced dementia and their caregivers. The other program was the Penn South Program for Seniors, the senior center of the Penn South Cooperative housing complex.

For seven years, graduate art therapy student interns and I offered sessions at Lenox Hill and Penn South. The students rotated annually, so through the years, the program was lucky to have gained abundantly from the creative energy of nearly 20 student interns. They were encouraged to draw from their own interests and observations to craft new ways to engage older participants. For example, when developing a mosaic project, students considered how the independent-living Penn South participant would engage with and benefit from the project, as well as how the same project could be adapted for a CARE participant with advanced dementia and limited mobility. What adaptations would need to be made to the art-making tools and process? What are the anticipated outcomes and goals? Would they be similar or different, and why? This helped to develop in the students the flexibility and ability to adjust quickly to the needs of a dynamic group therapy environment.

For each idea, students created a written protocol that addressed the goals, purpose, anticipated outcome, and process. As a result, the NYU CATS program amassed a thick binder of arts-engagement ideas. Some were very popular and successful and used over and over, sometimes with tweaks or additions. Others didn't work out so well, but we learned from them. Over the years, we became confident in what was likely to be most effective, beneficial, and enjoyable for both the Lenox Hill and Penn South groups. Many of those arts engagement ideas are presented in this book, and all of them inform my understanding of art therapy with older people.

Lenox Hill CARE

The CARE program served older people across New York City. Most participants lived at home on the East Side of Manhattan in the fulltime care of family and caregivers, who accompanied them to the program daily. Originally designed as a respite program for caregivers, the CARE program evolved to provide older people with dementia a safe and enjoyable place to spend the day among peers. Led by program director Elizabeth Hartowicz, this person-centered program assured each attendee that they belonged.

Each day began with a refreshment period for coffee, cookies, and donuts, which lasted up to an hour, since people arrived at their own pace. For those with dementia, dressing, bathing, eating, taking medicine, and ambulation can often take hours. Add in the snarling New York traffic, and the arrival time had to be fluid. The vibe was upbeat, as attendees were greeted joyfully by Elizabeth and other staff, volunteers, and peers. Conversation around the table might range from newsy to personal, but there was always laughter. Elizabeth had a wonderful way of finding the humor in most situations and was masterful at creating meaningful conversation out of the often disjointed or offbeat remarks.

On the days we offered art therapy sessions, our program began after the morning coffee hour and lasted until lunch arrived, which was supposed to be noon. However, lunch would at times arrive early, prompting a hurried cleanup of artwork, art materials, artist's hands, and the tables on which lunch would be served. Elizabeth had generous friends who were delighted to share their creative talents with the CARE participants. For example, two pianists alternated daily concerts after lunch. I encouraged my students to stay beyond our sessions from time to time just to witness the power of music with this group. While participants might be disengaged or even fall asleep during our group, when the music started, the same people could be observed hopping up out of their wheelchairs, dancing, and singing the words to songs of their youth. Other days, Elizabeth might "take them on a vacation" whereby a destination would be the theme of the day. The group watched videos or photos of places some might have been to or knew of, sparking excited conversation. Food from that region would be included as well. Sometimes participants would assist in preparing it, but always they would enjoy the smells and flavors of the food as it was prepared in the room. This multi-sensory "travel" experience was inclusive and joyful.

At times there were longer projects. Elizabeth directed participants in a rousing production of *My Fair Lady*, an endeavor that was the culmination of a year of casting, rehearsing, character development, set and costume design, and coping with the endless cycle of replacements for cast members who became ill or died.

Penn South

The Penn South Program for Seniors (PSPS) is a well-established centerpiece of Penn South, officially known as Mutual Redevelopment Houses, Inc., a cooperative housing community located in the Chelsea neighborhood of Manhattan. Serving as the hub of social services, PSPS links residents with supportive social work and nursing services to foster ongoing independent living. PSPS also offers a wide range of classes and lectures for senior residents, as well as discount theater tickets and transportation. At the time of our partnership agreement, PSPS's programming was significantly reduced due to funding losses, so the NYU CATS free-of-charge weekly art therapy program was a welcome addition.

Initially, we offered two separate sessions, an open studio art session available to all and a second specifically for physically frail elders. While the open studio was well attended from the beginning, the program for the physically frail was poorly attended. It took place in a large communal space on the first floor of one of the buildings in the large complex, but this location was inaccessible for those needing the dedicated assistance of a caregiver to bring them to the program. Eventually, the open studio was the only one we offered.

Over the course of seven years, we had a roster of more than 50 people, with a stable of 20 or so artists who were regular attendees. Some had been professional artists, like Ernie, who painted movie and theater posters, and Naomi, who was a celluloid artist for popular cartoons. However, most participants were either nonprofessional artists or had little to no experience in art. Although each was a resident of Penn South, most attendees did not know one another prior to attending the studio. The housing complex is quite large, occupying six New York City blocks, so their being unacquainted with one another was not unusual, but the fact that all the participating artists were from Penn South was a factor in creating the deep sense of community that this group developed.

Penn South was billed as an open art studio, and "therapy" did not appear in the advertisements. This was by design, as I worried that the term would deter people or mislead them about the nature of the program; many PSPS elder residents were not raised with arts and therapy. While I was careful in how the program was advertised, at the same time, I believed it did have much to offer therapeutically. I did make it clear, however, that I was an art therapist and art therapy instructor at New York University and that the students with me were studying art therapy.

My students and I struggled with the definition, scope, and practice of art therapy in this open studio setting with older people, as it was different than what any of us had learned in graduate school, which was centered primarily around working with children, teens, and adults in schools and hospitals and outpatient settings. Very little was written about art therapy with older people, and what was available problematized the symptoms of aging. This lack of resources required us to draw from knowledge and inspiration outside the realm of art therapy. Creative aging was emerging, and leaders such as Susan Perlstein's work with Elders Share the Arts, for example, helped us to frame our work in art therapy with older people.

Initially, the students and I were cautious about offering too much assistance and unwanted suggestions. We offered ideas to attendees and demonstrated various art media as we gradually acquired a broad assortment of supplies housed in a locked, walk-in storage closet. Students experimented with offering the same ideas for art making to both the Care and PSPS program participants, with significant adaptations. At PSPS, the offering was merely a suggestion since the artists frequently had their own ideas of how to spend their time and energy. Friendships developed, and ideas were shared. The creative energy was palpable each week, lifting us up from a dreary, poorly lit, echoing, industrial-sized multipurpose room to an environment where the sunlight and trees seemed to make their way through the narrow windows, music transported us, and laughter and sharing sharpened the meaningful connections being made.

Examples of Creative Aging Programs

The MultiMedia Arts Project

The Multimedia Arts Project at the Jewish Community Housing for the Elderly (JCHE) was an arts in health program funded twice by a National Endowments for the Arts ArtWorks grant. JCHE partnered with Lesley University's Institute for Arts and Health to deliver the project, which enabled 1,500 low-income older adults living in JCHE's affordable independent non-denominational housing to engage in creative arts opportunities that promoted healthy aging. Led by expressive therapists and teaching artists, participants explored diverse artistic disciplines and creative modalities specifically adapted to build community, enhance cross-cultural appreciation, increase self-esteem, improve motor and cognitive skills, and promote meaningful social connections among older adults.

The project was a time-limited offering to residents of four separate apartment buildings and included art and music-making workshops, mural-building, drama, dance, creative movement, and storytelling. Some programs were offered as a single event while others were a 6–8 week series. Each built a sense of community through enhanced modes of communication and expression, creating an inclusive environment that allowed participants to engage with the arts – especially those limited by mobility, language, or disability. A mixed-method evaluation of the program documented positive outcomes, including improvement in community livability.

Some workshops included the Playback Theater, which was very popular among residents; their feedback indicated that the actors gave voice to the lived experience of JCHE residents, who tended to be isolated from each other due to language and other differences. This workshop helped to connect this diverse community. Over a period of several months, a community mural – a vibrant representation of those who live at JCHE – was created in two residences.

Collaborating with a fitness professional, I offered a movement and art group. The fitness professional guided residents through a challenging sequence of stretches and dynamic movements beginning with chair exercises, with lively music and encouragement as the backdrop. With participants enlivened by the movement, the group then shifted to art-making. They were asked to replicate their favorite movement from the exercise portion in line, shape, and color, using the kinetic movements and gestures they had just made.

A program evaluation of the MultiMedia Arts Project found that residents developed a rich sense of belonging, connection, and community through engaging in the arts activities. This was evidenced by increased movement and gesturing toward other participants, by statements referencing connection, and by participant surveys. Residents were enthusiastic participants in the program, and creative expression proved to be an excellent way for them to communicate their feelings. Residents also self-reported and demonstrated expressions of joy and gratitude for the opportunity to engage with their peers through the arts. They generously expressed their appreciation to the teaching artists as well as to each other.

The MultiMedia Arts Project enlivened the JCHE residences, and both residents and staff expressed interest in having an ongoing program. Although this program was time-limited and tied to grant funding, it has led to ongoing programming with art, music, and dance/movement therapists who continue to engage the residents of JCHE.

Arts for the Aging

Another example of a creative aging program is Arts for the Aging, a social service organization that serves older adults and caregivers in greater Washington, DC, with innovative, multidisciplinary arts engagement aimed at health improvement and life enhancement. Founded in 1988 by sculptor Lolo Sarnoff to promote self-worth and independence, Arts for the Aging has developed some of the best arts engagement programs for older people in the nation. Arts for the Aging's faculty, consisting of professional artists trained in creative aging methodology, engage older people with mild to moderate physical or cognitive challenges in visual art, music, theater, dance, creative writing, and more. It runs in adult day programs, senior centers, community centers, elder residence communities, and museums. These programs engage older people in meaningful artistic expression that has been shown to improve mood, communication with peers, and imagination (Arts for the Aging, 2020). The person-centered programs offer a cost-effective means to "minimize aging-related physical and cognitive impairments, and contributes to better physical, intellectual and emotional health" (Arts for the Aging, 2020).

Many of Arts for the Aging's programs utilize multiple art forms. For example, the Connecting through Creativity program uses visual arts, poetry, story, and movement to evoke imagination while exposing participants to the work of artists and poets. In one program, Co-OPERAtion, led by a professional singer, participants experience an interactive performance of operatic music with costume, singing, moving, and storytelling. Another program, Digital Storytelling, is an intergenerational program pairing students with older adults to learn digital photography and videography. Intergenerational participants learn about the lives of one another and film a video. In response to the pandemic, Arts for the Aging developed and now offers live, telephonic, pre-recorded, heART Kits, and caregiver/training programs, all customizable and multidisciplinary. The heART Kits address the digital divide, recognizing that not everyone has access to computers and reliable wifi, and client partners deliver, in person, a visual art kit along with a meal. Arts for the Aging collaborated with the Smithsonian Institute's National Museum of African Art and National Portrait Gallery. The programs have expanded the museums' "artistic modalities to inspire music-making and dance-making evoked by the art and the stories they illuminate" (Arts for the Aging, 2020).

One especially notable Arts for the Aging program is Quicksilver Dance Company. Quicksilver is a professional dance troupe comprising people aged 60 years and over, many of them octogenarians. Quicksilver also provides participatory improvisational dance programs at community and residential care settings throughout the Washington DC area. This includes adult day centers, senior centers, community centers, memory cafes, affordable housing communities, assisted living and memory care facilities, nursing homes, museums and cultural institutions, and now at-home online programs. Founded by Nancy Havlik in 1997, Quicksilver uses dance and music to "begin a conversation" with participants, who engage through their own creative movement responses (Hyatt, 2017).

The National Endowment for the Arts has recognized Arts for the Aging's highly acclaimed Teaching Artist Institute as a leader in creative aging programs nationwide. In this institute, dedicated teaching artists offer training to professional artists in Arts for the Aging's best practices. Training is also offered to family members and caregivers who wish to learn about creative aging and engage with their loved ones through the arts.

Concluding Thoughts

The development of the creative economy and the workforce of art therapists and teaching artists is essential for the growth of these fields and their ability to meet the needs of an enormous segment of the population who can benefit from their services. In particular, assumptions that teaching artists (and artists in general) are volunteers and/or not paid as professionals must be dispelled. Art therapists and teaching artists are professionals whose artistic and educational skill sets, specialized training, and experience are valuable assets.

There are many avenues for engagement with older people through the arts. The past 15 years have seen a notable increase in arts engagement programs, as the connection between the arts and health and well-being continues to be substantiated through research guided by recommendations from a federal taskforce, including the National Endowment for the Arts and the National Institutes of Health (NEA, 2013). Art therapists themselves have documented, researched, and published their work with older people, significantly bolstering the body of research on this topic. Nevertheless, a great need and opportunity remain, with many older people ready, available, and in need of arts engagement programs like those described above. I sincerely hope that the momentum gained in the last decade and a half will lead to a future where arts engagement is available to all older people who wish to benefit from its proven ability to improve their health and well-being.

References

Arts for the Aging. (2020). https://Arts for the Agingarts.org/

Bennington, R., Backos, A., Harrison, J., Etherington Reader, A., & Carolan, R. (2016). Art therapy in art museums: Promoting social connectedness and psychological well-being of older adults. *The Arts in Psychotherapy, 49*, 34–43. https://doi-org.ezproxyles.flo.org/10.1016/j.aip.2016.05.013

Cantu, G., & Fleuriet, K. J. (2018). Making the ordinary more extraordinary: Exploring creativity as a health promotion practice among older adults in a community-based professionally taught arts program. *Journal of Holistic Nursing, 36*(2), 123–133. doi:10.1177/0898010117697863

Cohen, G., Perlstein, S., Chapline, J., Kelly, J., Firth, K., & Simmens, S. (2007). The impact of professionally conducted cultural programs on the physical health, mental health, and social functioning of older adults: 2-Year results. *Journal of Aging, Humanities and the Arts, 1*, 5–22.

Hanna, G.H., Noelker, L. S., Bienvenu, B. (2015). The arts, health, and aging in America: 2005–2015. *The Gerontologist, 55*(2), 271–277. doi:10.1093/geront/gnu183

Henley, D. (1995). A consideration of the studio as therapeutic intervention. *Art Therapy: Journal of the American Art Therapy Association, 12*(3), 188–190.

Hyatt, A. (2017). Creative aging with Quicksilver. *International Journal of Creativity and Human Development, 5*(1). https://www.creativityjournal.net/contents/issue-5-creative-aging-in-the-usa/item/357-creative-aging-with-quicksilver

Kramer, E. (1971). *Art therapy with children.* Chicago: Magnolia Street Publishers.

Kramer, E. (1986). The art therapist's third hand: Reflections on art, art therapy, and society at large. *American Journal of Art Therapy, 24*(3), 71–86.

Livingston, L., Fiterman Persin, G., & Del Signore, D. (2016). Art in the moment: Evaluating a therapeutic wellness program for people with dementia and their care partners. *Journal of Museum Education, 41*(2), 100–109.

Naumburg, M. (1950). *Introduction to art therapy.* New York: Teachers College Press.

Nea (2013). https://www.arts.gov/sites/default/files/Arts-and-Aging-Building-the-Science.pdf

Timm-Bottos, J. (2016). Beyond counseling and psychotherapy, there is a field. I'll meet you there. *Art Therapy, 33*(3), 160–162. doi:10.1080/07421656.2016.1199248

6   Identity, Connection, and Motivation

"Being with this wonderful group of interesting and talented people has opened a new and wonderful interest in art for me which I never had before."
– Ray

Early in my career, I firmly believed that the power of art therapy was in the artwork, that the truth of a person could be discovered in imagery. Trained from a psychodynamic perspective, I held earnestly to these initial goals. But over time, I have learned that while the work holds embedded meaning, what is most important in work with many older people stems from the art-making process as well as the artwork, through which the artist is seen, supported, and celebrated.

My practice has also shifted over time, from psychodynamic training to a person-centered approach. I can't hope to reverse memory loss through art therapy; in most cases, dementia is caused by irreversible organic changes in the brain. Attempting to "fix" memory only frustrates and disempowers the person one is attempting to fix. It is more effective to alter the environment for that person so that it suits their bandwidth and ability. When I work with a person who has dementia, I support the abilities they continue to have rather than attempt to retrieve those they have lost. The same is true, for example, of people who are grieving a loved one or feeling the loss of home, independence, or more. It is impossible to bring back a loved one who has died or restore the lost capabilities that had allowed a person to live independently. What I can do is to help them regain their balance and adjust to the loss and its consequences by strengthening their sense of self and supporting their resilience.

Using the embodied, person-centered approach described by Kontos and Naglie (2007), I see the person before me for who they are and the life they have lived. This lens is better suited to supporting and enhancing the capacities and strengths of older people. Person-centered care focuses on an individual's needs rather than their illness and seeks to enhance their strengths. As illustrated by Ahessy (2017) and Love and Pinkowitz (2013), psychosocial interventions and communication are the main focus of person-centered care of older people, particularly those with dementia. The goals of practice presented in this chapter embrace this tenet of the person-centered approach to therapy.

Goals

Years of hands-on work as an art therapist, observation of older people making art, and in-depth research with older artists like Rose, Adeena, and Marcia (see chapter 2), have led me to my current understanding of the goals that art therapists and teaching artists can use to frame and orient their work. Essentially, older people have let me know that what they are searching for is a life worth living. One individual is trying to maintain social connections, another their sense of fulfillment or satisfaction, yet another using the transcendence of age to develop an aspect of self that the vicissitudes of life prevented them from realizing earlier. In some cases, they are individuals who want to explore art-making for the first time or to continue their practice. In other cases, they are people with mild to severe dementia who benefit from a space and experience designed just for them. It is important to keep in mind the unique needs of each person. In considering the infinitely various experiences of older people, we must take into account that they approach their art and aging differently.

The principles outlined below – development of artist identity, connection, and motivation (Stephenson, 2013) – are the three main goals in my work with older people in art therapy (see Table 6.1 Goals).

Promote Development of an Artist Identity

Mary had an enduring artist identity, which she leaned on when coping with the death of her husband and her advancing macular degeneration. She had recently been widowed when she began to attend the open art studio. She was losing vision rapidly and wanted to prepare herself for blindness. A lifelong artist, Mary had taken some art courses but was not a professional artist. She came to the open art studio with the hope that she would figure out a way to make art as a blind person, and so my

Table 6.1 Goals

Goals
Promote Development of Artist Identity Foster Connection Instill Motivation

students and I explored some various materials that she might consider working with. Early in our work together, Mary drew with Sharpie markers, as they had bold, vibrant colors and she was slightly able to see the bold lines on the paper. Her drawings were abstract, colorful, moving lines of images that she had in her mind and memory. However, Mary was struggling with trying to re-create on paper what something looked like in her mind. Needless to say, she was frustrated.

Recognizing that drawing with the Sharpies was not the right path for her, my student interns and I began exploring different kinds of clay media. She didn't like the idea of her hands getting dirty with traditional clay, so we introduced plasticine, an oil-based, non-drying modeling medium that is typically used for casting models. She tried hard to manipulate the plasticine into various shapes that were appealing to her and made several forms but found the dense consistency of the plasticine too difficult to manipulate; it requires some heat in the hands in order to soften, and manipulating it effectively demands hand strength or the use of sculpting tools. Given the difficulty of working with this medium, Mary abandoned plasticine.

A traditional terra-cotta or air-drying clay was the next likely possibility, given that these media were softer and easier to work with, but Mary was no longer interested in anything clay-like. Of her own accord, she began making larger sculptures out of recycled materials. For example, she took a soup can, painted it, put legs on it, and made a series of humorous farm animals.

While exploring various media on her own at home, she began playing with the notion of switching art forms altogether and expressed interest in taking guitar lessons. After a while, abandoning the guitar, she expressed interest in working in a more flexible kind of clay, and so we offered her an air-drying clay option, since we did not have a kiln. This clay had a dark terra-cotta color and felt like a typical firing clay, with a texture soft to the touch. Almost immediately, Mary was able to manipulate it into forms that made sense to her. She had a strong understanding of composition, and it was really important to her to create a work that had a defined composition, and was both thematically and aesthetically compelling. But lacking vision, these factors needed to be something she could accomplish through touch.

Mary proceeded to make a series of sculptural designs that resembled an amphitheater with layered elements, like the Sydney Opera House. She said that she could touch these elements and very clearly understand what was happening in the form. She imagined that they were visually interesting, and I agreed – they commanded attention and played delightfully and purposefully with the negative space.

Mary began her work with us full of motivation to continue her engagement in the arts. Her creative capacity was strong, and I believe it probably had been throughout her life. She was using her creative abilities and her creative sensibilities to cope with two major losses, and she recognized that continuing to make art was absolutely vital for her well-being. She was a woman with a great deal of agency who took it upon herself to figure out how she could adapt to her new situation. In the face of loss, Mary realigned her life and drew on her assets to continue to live a life worth living.

Our role as therapists was to support Mary's exploration and her successes and failures along the way. We gently offered options, but gave her space to experiment and decide for herself what was working. The other open studio artists provided support as well. They were a community of people with whom she could identify, as many of them were also widowed, and some were also coping with vision loss.

Her story highlights an important point about this work: The goal is not to teach skills so that a person becomes a skilled or professional artist but rather to support development of the capacity and courage for artistic expression. To do this, art must first be demystified, relieved of the false notion that it belongs only in museums and art galleries and has to meet elite standards. My role as an art therapist is to encourage the exploration of art materials and the connections between feelings and thoughts and their expression through visual art media. The expectation is never to make a pretty picture or one that is worthy of exhibition – it is to unlock a new pathway to self-understanding and self-expression. As Mimi told me, "I am 88 years old, and I am learning new things about myself through art!"

Indeed, identity was a profound theme that continually emerged in my research with older women artists (Stephenson, 2010). Art and identity are intimately intertwined; considering oneself an artist gives permission and means to express oneself and discover ways of relating and interacting with the world that were previously not known or identified.

Foster Connection

Art-making, as well as attending art classes and visiting museums and galleries, are valuable for making social connections, and a primary goal in nearly all my work with older people is to foster connection – to others and to themselves.

From time to time, my student interns and I would offer a theme or question for the open studio artists to consider. (It was their choice to pursue it or proceed with their own ideas.) In one session, we asked them to consider their support system, and most were keen to explore this topic.

Ernie was a 98-year-old man who had been a professional graphic artist. He painted himself in *Painting theSistine* held aloft by his three children as he paints a large ceiling (Figure 6.1 Painting the Sistine). Ernie had been struggling with the decision to relocate to live closer to one

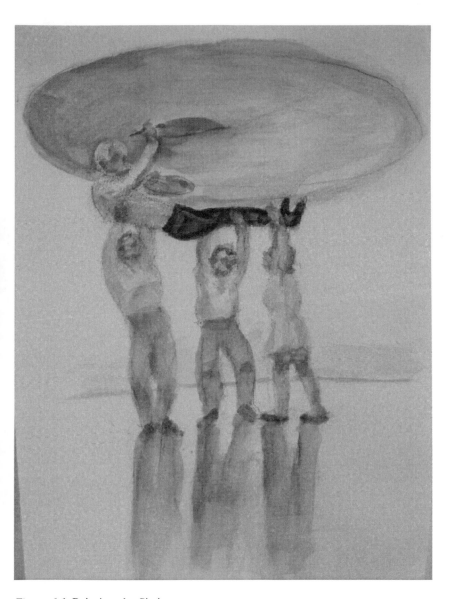

Figure 6.1 Painting the Sistine.

of his children. He was reluctant to leave behind his life in New York, but recognized he needed their help more and more. Similarly, Tony painted his children and grandchild. Although his family lived nearby, Tony had also discussed needing their help in order to continue to live independently. Gloria painted herself at the doctor's office – perhaps an unlikely image of support; yet, it made sense given her recent medical problems and the countless hours she had spent there. Maureen painted a woman at the grocery store. She described how she ordered her groceries for delivery once a week. She spoke with the same person each time but had never met her. One week, Maureen did not call and place the order, and the woman called to see if she was okay.

While the art-making itself is filled with value and meaning, stepping back from it, observing it, reflecting on it, and discussing it with others is perhaps the most important aspect of facilitation in a visual arts realm. In our display and discussion of the artwork at the close of the session, this common experience of needing connection and support was shared with great honesty and empathy among the group participants. During the art sharing, participants' work can be witnessed, acknowledged, and honored by others. The common experience of taking the risk to make art is there on display in the body of work exhibited. It is in this phase that an older artist might have an important realization about themselves, either through their own artwork or that of others. In this way, the closing phase of the session supports both the development of community and a deeper connection to oneself.

There are many ways that connection to others can be lost. Finding ways to bridge these losses is a main focus of much of my work. I approach this by helping my client identify the connections and assets they do have. This strength-based approach builds upon what is already there. In my view, that is the best and, at times, the only way to approach growth.

Many studies show that being connected to others is an integral part of health and well-being. In our younger lives, we have numerous threads of connection related to the multiple roles we play. In fact, it isn't uncommon to seek *dis*connection as a reprieve from the stress of being constantly connected – by email, social media, text, phone, and our in-person responsibilities as partners, parents, caregivers, employees, citizens, and more. And yet, with advanced age comes a loosening of these connections – by choice, or retirement, or relocation, or selective socializing; by death, or bodily changes like vision loss or frailty that make mobility much more difficult. While some argue that it is natural to disconnect in older adulthood, it is important to assess whether that disconnection is by choice or circumstance. Most often, it is the latter.

A common problem for many older people, social isolation is linked to loneliness, depression, and physical illness. Social isolation occurs when a person does not have the amount or kind of contact with other people that they want. They want a more robust life, they want more connection with people. Social connection is not only a vital component of feelings of satisfaction, but it also contributes to personal growth, increased self-esteem, and an increased sense of purpose.

Instill Motivation

Marina was in her late eighties when she began attending the open art studio while continuing to work one day per week as an accountant. She said she wished to learn how to paint – a skill she never learned as a child. Other than training miniature bonsai, she claimed she had never "been creative." Marina had severe arthritis in her legs, which made it difficult for her to walk; yet, she attended the art studio nearly every Monday for several years. She was eager to learn and frequently asked for demonstrations. Lifelong learning was clearly an ongoing aspiration for her.

Slowly but surely, Marina gained basic mastery over a range of drawing and painting techniques and media, and was curious about the mixed media works others were creating. Eventually, she began experimenting with found materials, assembling them into small three-dimensional pieces. Sometimes we offered Marina ideas as a place to begin, but increasingly, she worked from her own list of ideas generated during the week. For example, while talking on the telephone, she drew a long, spiraling doodle that represented the phone cord, which gave her all sorts of ideas to explore. I was impressed that she was so eager and thought about this during the week as if it were homework. She spent a lot of time talking to the other participants and paid attention to and learned from what other people were doing. She often told me, "I never knew I would learn so much about myself at this age! By making art in this class, I am learning about parts of myself I never knew were there."

Our role as leaders was to teach her the skills she requested, but it was also to support her motivation to attend the weekly open art studio, engage with her peers, and deepen her artistic expression. We recognized that each week she took a risk by making art and sharing it. Over the course of several years, her skills became better, but more importantly, her motivation pushed her to keep developing those skills alongside others in the community. I'm not sure she would have made art on her own in the same way.

Art was a connection in several areas of Jeremy's life. At one point, he had been a high school art teacher, and later he offered art classes to older adults in the community. He frequently attended the open studio sessions, where he skillfully drew portraits of himself and others with graphite, acrylic, and watercolors. Just shy of 100 years old, Jeremy told me he was always thinking about tomorrow and ideas for the future. In the open studio, he experimented with new media and depicting the human form, pushing to express himself in new ways. His artistry was ever-expanding and reaching into new areas yet unexplored. He exemplified how the arts can motivate a person to dream about tomorrow, share ideas with others, and find joy.

Several of these sketches highlight people with a sustained identity as an artist and thus more inherent motivation to make art. But an art therapy or creative aging program must still meet their needs and match their abilities, as it must for all attendees. If our understanding of a person's interest and abilities is incorrect, the experience we are offering is likely to not only be misaligned with their needs, but it could also be harmful or even dangerous. Certainly, it will not be joyful or spark motivation in them to return for more. And so, in order to achieve our goal, we must ensure that participants are set up to experience success, meaningfulness, and joy. The next three chapters will provide details about how to do this by exploring how a program should be structured, the process of engagement, the selection of art media, and considerations when working with people who have dementia.

The literature on creativity and aging, art therapy, and its clinical practice often focuses on the loss of physical faculties associated with age, such as eyesight and mobility. Changes to or loss of physical capabilities are prevalent among older adults I have worked with, impacting their lives in various ways. However, I have observed that motivation is a key factor in their resilience and adaptation to these changes, including the motivation to continue to make art. Marcia, described in depth in chapter 2, had been severely limited by chronic fatigue syndrome, which slowed down her creative process and limited her ability to leave her house. While one would expect this to have had a negative impact on her work, she insisted that art-making gave her a reason to get up and get to work every day, despite extreme fatigue.

People are driven by expectations. But more often than not, what feels good and enjoyable inspires action (and conversely, what doesn't feel good evokes uncomfortable emotions like frustration and anger). Of course, some people find themselves in an art therapy session because participation is required, but generally, participation is by choice. Regardless of what brought participants, I try to make their experience not only meaningful but joyful if possible. At the same time, I am aware that frustration, disappointment, fear, and a host of uncomfortable feelings are likely to emerge. Ultimately, my aim is to offer a meaningful experience that will motivate people to invest deeply in the process. I do this by helping them give life to their feelings through visual media.

References

Ahessy, B. (2017). Song writing with clients who have dementia: A case study. *The Arts in Psychotherapy.* https://doi-org.ezproxyles.flo.org/10.1016/j.aip.2017.03.002

Kontos, P. C., & Naglie, G. (2007). Bridging theory and practice: Imagination, the body, and person-centred dementia care. *Dementia, 4,* 549.

Love, K., & Pinkowitz, J. (2013). Person-centered care for people with dementia: A theoretical and conceptual framework. *Generations: Journal of the American Society on Aging, 37*(3), 23–29.

Stephenson, R. C. (2010). *The creative experience of women: Art making and old age*. ProQuest Dissertations & Theses (PQDT). Web. 6 July 2012.

Stephenson, R. C. (2013). Promoting wellbeing and gerotranscendence in an art therapy program for older adults. *Art Therapy: Journal of the American Art Therapy Association, 30*(4), 151–1581.

7   Structure and Process

"It is a vivifying, enlivening experience every week, a curative for most ills and a relaxant and relevant relief from the rest of the world." – Louisa

Cultivating a space where creativity can flourish is essential. This chapter explores how the concept of liminal space sets up the opportunity for play and discovery. Building from there, physical considerations of the space, as well as pacing and division into segments, frame the overall structure of an art-making session, whether it is art therapy or a creative aging program. The unique benefits of making art in the presence of others, as well as the benefits of working one on one, are also explored. The chapter concludes with the joyful celebration of the art exhibition.

How I Understand Art-Making

When I set out to make art, I choose the material I wish to work with but usually don't have a plan, theme, or vision for what I want to make. Rather, I play with the material, letting the brush strokes play freely, the color drip unexpectedly. I rejoice in the surprises that emerge in front of me; they invite me to engage in a visual dialog. Will I reply to the surprise or let it be? Playing with the media breathes life into the process; it is allowed space to be what it wants to be (e.g., wet paint dripping, heavy clay slumping, hard pencil scratching). I don't begin as a master of the picture. I am co-creator, allowing the dynamic properties of the media to be themselves, inviting me to play with them, push them, challenge them. After some time, I begin to notice patterns in the dialog and, maybe later, a theme. At this point, I step into a more dominant role in the dialog, making a more concerted effort to harness the media, to push it where I want to go. Ultimately, the artwork has been created from my hand, guided by my choices, but it all began from a playful interaction with the visceral qualities of the media.

Often, I make art to music. The music guides my work, especially in the beginning, when I am not sure what to do. Music has the power to quickly influence my mood, set the stage, and take me back to experiences I haven't thought of for decades. Sometimes the tunes stay in the background as I focus on the image or my thoughts. But sometimes, the music reaches deep into my gut and grabs hold. When that happens, my art is strongly tethered to the feelings it evokes.

I have always enjoyed music by Neil Diamond. He has been an artist in the backdrop of my life rather than on the main stage, and yet, while listening to Neil Diamond while making art one day, I was astounded by the depth of my connection to very old memories and feelings, as his velvety, soulful voice guided my hand as I pushed and pulled my paintbrush. Playing with the visceral qualities of the paint, powered by this soundtrack, I found myself transported back to my childhood. Flashes of afternoons spent at the town pool with "Shiloh" playing to the crowd over crackling speakers rushed forth. "America" and other songs from the *Jazz Singer* movie soundtrack made me think about how, as young girls, my sister and I bristled at joining our mother at the movies to see the film. Despite our complaints that we had no interest in hearing "jazz," we went and saw the film. And ... it was transformative! We fell in love with the story and especially the music. We bought the soundtrack, and for a long time afterward, we performed *Jazz Singer* singalongs in our living room.

I hadn't thought about that for a very long time. But as I sat quietly painting in unusually careful detail, with Neil playing to my heart, the memory emerged, along with a range of very old feelings. Although it unboxed feelings of sorrow and deep hurt of that time in my life, which was shortly after my father died, the memory of our dancing lightheartedly to the *Jazz Singer* soundtrack made me realize, perhaps for the first time, that there were good times during those painful years, and that our house was often filled with music. I could not have willed that realization into existence. However, the kinesthetic and sensory components of the art media sparked feelings and, enhanced by music, they moved me deeper into memory, sensory, and emotional recall, all without talking or thinking explicitly about it. I tell you this story because it describes how art-making can help to connect older people – with and without dementia – to themselves. It is a powerful mechanism for life review and reminiscence, of course. But, day to day, it provides an opportunity to ignite and celebrate vitality in large and small ways.

My approach to working with older people is the same as my own art-making process. Rather than begin with a theme, idea, or goal in mind, I encourage people to begin with play and exploration. Not only is this a less threatening way to introduce art-making, which for many is intimidating, but it can be a more effective means of achieving the whole point of the process, which is to experience joy and reignite connections to self and others through new pathways, with their endless permutations.

The Transitional Space

Psychotherapist Donald Winnicott (1971) wrote about the mother/child attachment and how the mother, through trust, consistency, and encouragement, creates a safe space within which the child can play, explore, and learn. As an entity separate from the mother, slowly and through experimentation, the child explores the world through touch, smell, movement, and play. Winnicott named this imaginary realm the "transitional space," a sort of intermediate area of experiencing, where a person feels protected by imaginal boundaries in order to feel free on the inside to explore and test themselves.

The space in which older people come together with an art therapist or teaching artist can also serve as a holding environment in which this transitional space can exist. In this way, the art therapist or teaching artist creates a boundary within which the older person can play and find success and joy. The facilitator constructs this holding environment by creating a set of rules and a structure for the session, including use of the physical space and art materials. When you think about the life of somebody with Alzheimer's disease, for example, who is constantly living in a world that might now seem confusing or frightening, the opportunity for that person to experience an environment that is tailored or suited to these limitations is valuable. Such a space is geared toward creating a sense of emotional as well as physical safety. The art therapy session can be crafted not only to eliminate stressors such as questions that require memory – those starting with "do you remember ...," for example – but also to tap into the vibrant inner life of an older person, even if they have advanced Alzheimer's disease. Creating an environment in which that person succeeds in what they do allows them to feel successful and even joyful.

Ideally, arts engagement encounters take place in a dedicated art-making space. However, the reality is that the space made available for art-making often is used for a variety of purposes, including eating meals. This might mean that there is limited or no storage capacity for art supplies and nowhere to display or store artwork. Multi-use surfaces are usually not designed for heavy-duty art-making and instead are better suited for eating lunch, writing a note, or reading a book or magazine. Working in spaces where meals are served is particularly challenging, as the tables need to be thoroughly sanitized. Art media such as paint, glue, or clay can leave a significant amount of residue and require detailed cleaning. But despite adaptations to comply with the restrictions of the space, deeply meaningful experiences still occur.

In this regard, the quality of the interaction between therapist/artist, participant, and art-making is paramount. When the participant is seen, witnessed, known, and heard, the interpersonal attunement that occurs is therapeutic.

Following are two examples of how we worked with the outer environment and its limitations to create an environment for art-making for older adults.

Lenox Hill CARE

We were lucky to meet this group in a large church basement with old hardwood floors, interior brick walls, a small kitchen, a storage area, and plenty of tables and chairs. There was even a grand piano! Although the lighting was more ambient than bright, the space was easily adaptable to art-making, from table-top work to larger, floor-based work. The rectangular tables were large and sturdy and could be rearranged in large or small clusters as needed. Though there might be 6–12 participants per day, often an additional 6–12 staff, volunteers, caregivers, and interns were assisting. So, the space really needed to be appropriate for up to 24 people.

Often, we worked side by side with participants, the spacious room allowing us to move about fluidly without too much trouble or interruption. We worked around a cluster of tables and then moved the chairs across the room, where the art would be hung and participants seated in a semicircle to view their work. The kitchen was an invaluable water source for painting and cleaning. There was also ample storage to keep art supplies tucked away and completed artwork safely contained in folders for each person, laid flat so as not to bend or crease paper. Aside from the lighting, the only other limitations to the space were that it was used by other groups on the weekends, so nothing could be permanently displayed on the walls. In addition, its location far on the edge of Manhattan's East Side was difficult to reach by public transportation.

Eventually, the CARE program was moved to a very small space in a Lenox Hill Neighborhood House building, a space that was woefully inadequate for the program and its attendees. With most participants in wheelchairs, the fit around the table was tight, and there was little room for anyone to maneuver. It was difficult for staff and volunteers to help participants with their work. Seated elbow to elbow, we awkwardly maneuvered our arms, squeezing between participants in order to lend a hand. The art viewing also took place at the table, as there was not enough room to relocate. This put the artists at the far end of the table at a disadvantage in that they were less able to see the work on the wall or hear what was being said. We made adjustments to accommodate this setup, such as using a microphone and a large screen to project the image. Or, while seated around the table, artists held up their own work, one by one, so that it was more of a "moving gallery" discussion. Storage was very limited, so our range of supplies and the kinds of arts engagement activities we could try were limited. And without a sink, art preparation and clean up were more complicated. However, we became adept at planning for these sessions, staging art materials, and having additional materials on hand to change course as needed. Fortunately, there was a small piano at the back of the room, so the vibrant live music interludes continued. The benefits of this space, however, were that it was well lit, we were able to permanently display the artwork of participants, and the building had easier access to transportation, access to adjunctive senior services in the same building, greater proximity to the homes of attendees, and an accessible building design.

Penn South

Operating in the large community room on the ground floor of one of the Penn South apartment buildings was truly a gift. The space was easy to access by walker or wheelchair, with clean, wide paths leading through the courtyard right to the front door. We had access to an abundance of foldable long tables and chairs that could be arranged in any way fathomable. However, due to the fluorescent track lighting, we usually aligned the tables directly under the lights. There were large white plaster walls upon which we could tape our daily creations, with chairs seated before the "gallery" where enlivened conversations about the work grew in length and depth over the years. The room was equipped with a bathroom, including an additional slop sink. Because it was a multi-purpose room, it needed to be returned as it was at the end of each session; however, with plenty of storage, each artist had a large artist portfolio folder in which to keep their artwork.

The locations of art therapy and creative aging programs for older people varies widely. Nevertheless, for its ability to empower older people and encourage artistic identity, art therapy's open art studio model can be especially effective. Allen (1995) noted that the open art studio is an effort to "break down barriers and boundaries between people, creating compassion and empathy" (p. 166). Believing that art-making itself heals even without interpretation, she argues that the opportunity to witness the infectious energy that often exists in an art group allows genuine and long-lasting results to be achieved. Allen writes that "viewing the struggles of one another through art causes shifts of perception on a deep level. This occurs not so much in insight gained through discussion as in simple witnessing" (p. 166).

The Three Parts of a Session

My experiences working with groups of older people making art has been nothing short of profound. While the artwork itself can be a valuable catalyst to explore deep feelings in art therapy, the entire process from beginning to end is of great value: the coming together of the group, setting up, making, sharing, and departing. Each session can be divided into three parts – the introduction, art-making, and sharing and discussion.

The Introduction

Saying hello is in and of itself a ritual. I am grateful that those who come to my art group have wanted to expend the great deal of effort it took for them just to arrive. I try my best to greet each participant with enthusiasm, showing and telling them how much I value them and their presence in the group. Whether the plan for the day is an open studio where people are free to do what they want, or a more structured art process that requires demonstration, I introduce the session, what we will be doing, for how long we'll be making art, and at what time we will begin to clean up and transition to the art-viewing discussion. In some instances, it is important that I introduce myself and students or staff who are working with me, and, I ask participants to introduce themselves as well. I will also offer suggestions, materials, themes, or questions as a means to give inspiration. For groups that involve more structured instructions, I spend ample time describing the prompt and materials and demonstrating how to use them. From there, I may move around the room, from person to person, to offer hands-on assistance where needed or verbal support.

Of course, what brings us together is making art. But that is not all that we are doing. We are being together, socializing, and sharing little or large bits of our daily lives with each other. I have found it valuable to allow time at the beginning for people to talk to one another and get settled before launching into the plan for the day. These moments of social interaction really help people feel comfortable in the space, connecting at first in ways that feel safe. Small talk about the corner coffee store increasing its prices or the blooming dogwood trees can ease people into an unfamiliar situation – and for most people, making art is an unfamiliar situation.

Art-Making

Artists are both witness to the process of others and subjects of the same curiosity from their peers. I have the privilege of a vantage point that allows me to see the group process unfolding before me – to see, for example, the colors and themes of one artist wordlessly influencing someone sitting next to them or across the table. How validating it is when what we are doing is not only noticed by another but inspires their actions! I have noticed that people often feel unsure of themselves at the beginning of a session. Making art isn't something people often do as part of their regular life, and many equate making a picture with the evaluation of it. When I ask a person to make art with me, my request is often met with trepidation. However, when that person notices they are not alone in their caution, they feel more comfortable with their discomfort – and that leads to their becoming more emboldened.

As one person dips their toe into the cold water, the next tries, and then the next. It feels easier to take a risk when there are others around you doing the same. The shared experience of doing something challenging can be very powerful. Now these potential strangers have a bonding experience. This might not sound as bold or profound as climbing a mountain with an expedition or joining protesters marching for a just cause, but the core experience is the same. Such small experiences can change the course of a person's life ever so slightly and, over time, lead to significant change.

Imagine a person with dementia who is at times frightened by their world, which comes in and out of understanding, and who has become more and more withdrawn because of this uncertainly. If this person is able to feel successful while taking the harmless risk of painting a picture, they will not only feel better about themselves, but they will also be willing to try it again, and again, leading to more confidence and capacity in their new reality with dementia.

Sharing and Discussion

Janice was a core member of the art studio. She had been present from the beginning, and the art studio for her was as much a social event as it was a chance to make art. Janice expressed herself freely in a multitude of ways. Dressed in vibrant colors and patterns that frequently matched or contrasted with her dyed hair, Janice also felt comfortable taking risks in her artwork. Although she wasn't a technically skilled artist, she had a knack for colors that evoked powerful emotions. At one point, she revealed to the group that a tumor had been found near her eye and that she would endure a series of surgeries. Janice painted the tumor, expressing the headaches and visual distortions it caused with shape and color. Janice's "eye series" was difficult to "see" and to feel, knowing that our friend was suffering and afraid of the surgery and outcome. Both she and her artwork evoked deep feelings of care and concern in each of us. Her artwork served as a catalyst for discussion of her fears about impending surgery, as well as the disorientation and discomfort the tumor was causing. Often, the discussion circled around the artwork itself as a representation of her troubles. Fortunately, the surgery was successful, and Janice rejoined the group after several months of healing.

In the art therapy room, sharing our artwork is as valuable an experience as making it. I set aside ample time at the end of each session to discuss the work that has been produced, and whenever possible, I hang the art on a wall and seat people in front of it. If that isn't possible, we stay at the table and each person presents their work one by one. I invite the artist to say a few words about their work, followed by respectful comments from the audience. When we see our work at a distance, not only do we see it differently because of the altered vantage point, but we are also more emotionally detached from it. This distancing allows the artist to see the work as an entity separate from themselves. Artists have thoughts and feelings about their work, but by placing it in front of other viewers, it becomes part of their experience as well. The audience sees the work as an object with layered features, each connecting to it in their own way. At the same time, they are responding to its creator – the artwork becomes the artist's surrogate. There are multiple connective strands happening: between artists and artists, viewers and artists, artwork and artwork. An observer might see a group of older people clustered around drawings and paintings hanging on a wall, but I see the gathering as participants connecting to each other, to this group, and to themselves. The art-making and artwork are catalysts for this powerful phenomenon that is at the core of art therapy and creative aging.

Making Art in the Presence of Others

Much of the time, I do my own art practice alone in my studio. I am lucky to have a corner of the basement under a large window where I have an easel and table. There is ample shelving to store a variety of art supplies and floor space to move about comfortably. I try to ignore evidence of mice, the cold temperature, and the typical basement structural bones that detract from the aesthetic appearance of the space. But when I get into the work, those environmental details fade away, and I'm instead deeply focused. Although I am alone while working, I like to share my finished works and works-in-progress with my immediate family and select friends. I don't share to necessarily seek opinion or approval, but rather to share the novelty of something new being created. To me, art-making is a bit like magic. It surprises me, intrigues me, perplexes me, and confuses me. Art compels me to wonder the "what" and "why" of its existence.

There are many purposes and needs for making art. Solo work in a studio has its own purpose, but working alongside one or more other people has another. Social entities, we human beings need connection with others. When I am overscheduled with work, caring for my family, activities, social commitments, etc., I sometimes feel that what I need is disconnection. But I always need to be connected with and seen by others. This need is even more profound for older people. For many, retirement brings a reduction in connection with colleagues and a diminishing of their professional identity. Relocating to a new home, city, or state creates disconnection. Further, as people become less mobile they may become less able to engage in socializing, resulting in the very old sometimes being quite isolated. The Covid-19 pandemic has amplified isolation among elders to an alarming degree, particularly those residing in elder residences that have been locked down to visitors.

The Open Art Studio

Over the years, I have sharpened my understanding of what art therapy is and can be with older adults. The NYU CATS open studio group was initially designed to provide space and materials for older adults in the community to engage in art-making. Other than that, I did not have strict parameters about the format and was open to the needs and interests of the participants. The group attracted lifelong professional artists as well as those who had never made art before.

Despite the wide range of ability and training, it was remarkable how members of the group were able to support each other, to offer advice about technique and thoughtful feedback about content. The artists supported one another, offering generous praise and reserving criticism – phrased constructively – for the work. The group was powerful in this way, modeling the kind of comments they felt comfortable with. One new participant, at their first discussion, opened with criticism of the art only to return the following week, having learned from the others, to also show support for the artist's intent and experience. In this way, participants built a network of friendships that lived beyond the confines of the session. Participants met for coffee or lunch when the program was not in session, attended theater together, and went to galleries. They checked in on one another when a friend was ill and visited one another in the hospital.

According to Allen (1995), an art therapy group should focus on the concept that the primary art-making experience for all artists is self-expression, communication, feelings of wholeness. Likewise, examining the therapeutic effects of group participation, Flood and Phillips (2007) found that "group members may experience enhanced self-esteem, life satisfaction, improved problem-solving ability, and increased creativity. Moreover, a sense of universality and belonging can occur as peer relationships are developed" (p. 397). Working together in an open studio fosters empathy among group members and creates a more inspired and productive environment conducive to art-making. Additionally, attending an open studio can improve one's mood and feeling of self-esteem, statements echoed in the research of Wikström (2002) and Cohen et al. (2006).

I have observed that the older people who attended the open art studio were self-motivated and self-reliant. They looked for support from others rather than approval. An art therapy studio setting for older people should involve cautious and informed leadership on the part of the art therapist, within a supportive and enriching environment that is respectful of wisdom and life experience, while acknowledging the physical needs of the participants and adapting the space and tools accordingly. Participants are not looking for acknowledgment from their peers as much as they are for camaraderie and empathy – these are compelling sources of inspiration and safety for group members.

Jana

A petite older woman with short hair and a broad smile, Jana came to the open art studio and immediately sat down and began drawing. I was astounded that after only an hour Jana had created a larger than life-size self-portrait in charcoal. Often, people will draw self-portraits that are either life-size or smaller, but rarely larger than themselves. Jana selected the largest size paper we had available and was very clear about her choice of charcoal, using first vine charcoal and then block charcoal. When we hung up the art at the end of the session, Jana explained that the reason why she left one of the eyes unfinished was that she was legally blind in that eye. Many in the room were astonished by her sophisticated skill as an artist. She had depicted a strong likeness of herself. Others were amazed by her courage. Here is a person who, on her first day with a group that had existed for several years, jumped right in as if she had been a member for years. Others were curious about how she was able to create such a drawing when she was experiencing significant vision loss.

In subsequent weeks, Jana created a very large panorama of a childhood memory of herself and her sister at a summer camp. She had a creative way of approaching this drawing. With vine charcoal and a fragment of newsprint paper, she made sketches of parts of this image. The next week she would take another fragment of paper and make more sketches of another part of this memory. The vine charcoal was soft and impermanent, so it was easy for her to erase and redo her sketches. Watching Jana create this work over the course of several months, I struggled to see how the many sketches drawn on irregularly cut pieces of newsprint would fit together. It seemed that she was creating a fragmented giant puzzle. As she drew each week, she recounted various details of the experiences she and her sister shared as children. It seemed to me that the process of making this drawing was as important if not more important than the artwork itself. It was like a long drawn out telling of a beautiful story that meant so much to her. Eventually, she pieced the newsprint pieces together and redrew them with a more permanent, robust block charcoal over the vine charcoal. The image emerged with confidence and clarity! We framed the drawing and showed it in our annual art exhibition. This work, five feet long and two feet tall, was truly a masterpiece, a remarkable representation of how powerful art can be, and an example of creativity in old age. Jana was independent from start to finish, and her skill was in part the result of her lifelong involvement in the arts. But our work as a group leaders and the supportive open studio group environment offered her a chance for community, connection, laughter, and appreciation for her work. Jana was both coming to terms with the loss of vision as well as forming a connection with the group, which she needed but did not have.

The Benefits of Individual Work

The setup matters even in one-on one work between the therapist and client. The concepts of liminal and physical space are equally important in individual work when only the art therapist is present. Here, the power of the group is exchanged for the intimacy of personal attention. I worked with Judith in her home for 18 months, supporting her adjustment to life without vision.

Judith

I was introduced to Judith as someone I could help to make art again. Afflicted late in life with macular degeneration, a degenerative eye disease, she was legally blind by the time I met her. She was able to see little bits of color and light and shadow at the beginning of our work together, but that steadily declined. Judith had enjoyed throwing ceramic pots on the wheel and glazing them in blended colors but had given it up when she went blind, to her great dismay.

At the outset of our work together, she was unsure how she could make art again but was willing to give it a try. I was immediately impressed by her courage. Judith lived alone and was accustomed to leading an active and independent life. Becoming blind at nearly 90 years old, after living a long life with vision, was frightening and dramatically changed her quality of life. It robbed her of her ability to attend art classes and lectures, read books, go to the movies, choose a matching outfit from the closet, or cross a busy city street, among many other losses. And yet, she was learning how to arrange sets of clothing together to ensure they matched, she had phone sessions in which someone would read a book chapter to her, and she received white cane training so that she could leave her apartment on her own and safely navigate to her destination.

Our weekly work together involved a series of rituals, not unlike the structure of art therapy group work but reflective of the fact that our work was taking place in her home and was one to one. When I arrived at her orderly apartment, we greeted one another warmly and sat down at a wooden side table. The side table served as her workspace, a place where her artwork was safe and apart from more commonly used spaces. She stored her materials in bags underneath the table. In an effort to brighten the workspace, she placed a desk lamp on the end of the table. Over the months, we tried various kinds of lamps in the hope that brighter light would help her to see the work a little more. But it was futile, and eventually the lamp was removed.

Judith was not in the habit of making art in her apartment before she met me. Previously, she had worked in a ceramic studio where she could be messy and where she would eventually fire her pieces. She was careful about retaining few materials so as to not clutter the space or overwhelm herself.

My favorite ritual was the sharing of materials. Once seated at the side table, I joyfully opened a large bag full of items I had collected during the week in hopes that some of them would entice her. Some were those she specifically requested. Some were possibilities we had discussed, while others I chose on my own, curious to see her reaction. As I presented them one at a time, Judith held the material, feeling the texture, turning it over in her hands, and assessing it. She was decisive and let me know right away if she was interested in keeping the item. I was pleased to bring her these items and very much enjoyed hunting for new treasures for her throughout the week. My idea of possible art media expanded as I wandered through hardware stores looking for intriguing shapes, textures, forms, and possibilities.

At first, I assumed that because she was blind, it would be natural for her to experiment with the easily moldable, tactile clay. However, given that she had years of experience already working in clay, she was not interested in using a medium that she could no longer craft at the same level of control and intention she once had. So, at each session, we would discuss possible art media. She wanted to try working with red paper and pliable metallic surfaces like aluminum foil in hopes that she could still see some color and reflected light. Gradually, she let go of that notion and began relying on her sense of touch; we explored textured paper, fabric, and natural materials such as tree bark, beginning with two-dimensional collage.

Judith cut, glued, and arranged the materials into compositions, but she became increasingly frustrated by her inability to see what she was making. Gradually, she began to choose three-dimensional or highly textured objects, relying more on her sense of touch and less on her eyesight. Metal objects such as bolts, washers, wire, connectors, and plumbing hardware transformed into an elaborate sculpture. Symbolically, Judith's art had great meaning as the process of making this work marked an astounding parallel process to her development of special intelligence. Throughout the year, when she was working with me, she was learning to walk through the city using a white cane. Gradually she became more independent and ventured out alone for her walks, trusting the senses she retained. In the same way, by using spatial intelligence in making art, she gained confidence in her abilities. Soon, she began attending intergenerational ceramics classes at the senior center again and delighted in the new ways she could hand-build clay forms and use texture instead of glaze as a source for decorating.

The opportunity for us to work one on one in her home for more than a year was a luxury for both of us. She had my full attention during the session. I was amazed by Judith's courage and confidence. She was constantly experimenting, doing, undoing, and redoing. Among many things, I learned from Judith about perseverance and resilience in the face of the difficult loss of physical functioning late in life. I observed how her small successes were like bricks of confidence that grew into a strong wall of fortitude and strength. Judith's deep investment in her own process, with my support, enabled her to find the skill and confidence she needed to transition her identity and function as a blind woman.

Celebrating the Art: Exhibitions

In the spirit of promoting connection and artist identity, organizing an exhibition of participant artwork can be a joyful community celebration of elder artists. The paintings have dried and are framed, hanging on a clean, well-lit wall in a gallery or community space. Friends and family gather to view the collection of artwork of their loved one and their peers. There might be flowers on the tables with refreshments and stacks of postcards announcing the exhibition. The artists might be wearing a special garment or adornment for the occasion. Regardless, as the guests of honor, they will feel joyful in their accomplishments, and that sentiment will spread across the event.

The first annual NYU CATS art exhibition was a memorable one, setting the tone for seven more annual shows to follow. It is difficult to secure a professional art gallery, I learned early on. Space in New York City is often booked a year or more in advance. The next best option was to reserve an NYU gallery, but they, too, are booked far in advance, which is why the first exhibit was scheduled for early July – the first available date following the inaugural year of the program. July in New York is enjoyable when air conditioning is available on those muggy hot nights, but not so much when the a/c is broken and fans are insufficient to cool a room, especially with more than 60 people milling about, socializing, and looking at art. I was also concerned for the health and well-being of so many older people who traveled across town to attend.

The artwork had been carefully curated – each artist choosing two works to display. As per the project proposal, we had set aside funding to professionally frame the artwork – frames that I later re-matted and re-used for subsequent shows. An abundance of food and wine was carefully spread across black tablecloths, and tall flower bouquets balanced on the café tables. By the end of the night, every last cracker had been eaten and every drop of wine drunk – even the flowers made their way home with attendees! I was completely surprised by the sheer number of family and friends of the artists attending the exhibition. Clusters of people gathered around the artists as they posed in front of their artwork, which then morphed into group photos of all the exhibiting artists. The mood was joyful – the artists were clearly very proud of their work and its inclusion in this art exhibition. What I learned from this and every subsequent exhibit was how valuable this end-of-the-year culminating event was. It solidified participants' identity as an artist and deepened the NYU CATS community connection, but more than that, it shared that connection more broadly. How wonderful that friends and family had the opportunity to share such joy and inspiration!

Considerations for Dementia

An exhibition that is carefully curated and displayed and that values and celebrates the artwork can help reduce the stigma of aging and dementia. The artwork of people with dementia can be difficult to understand, as it might appear childish or incomplete. It is important to present to the viewers how the artwork represents the artist's presence and participation rather than focus on the mounting cognitive losses, which might reveal themselves as "amateurish." (Other words that might be used to describe the work if viewed conventionally are: *distorted, confused, simple,* or *fragmented*).

Unless witnessed directly, the true nature of the process of art-making is not obvious. Therefore, it is important to describe how the work was made, as these examples show:

> A true collaborator, Bonnie is a keen observer of those around her and allows her study to inspire and influence her work. Her painting process involves periods of working carefully on her own painting, then observing other artists. She also enjoys close student collaboration.

> Rena's creative process is as hypnotic as her paintings. She truly enjoys the process of painting, carefully exploring each color and pulling her brush along the paper as if on some great journey. All the while, Rena's outward enjoyment of the creative process inspires all those around her.

The opening of the show should be scheduled so that the artists can attend with their caregivers and family members. Family and caregivers are often surprised by the expressiveness of the artwork. During an exhibit of the CARE program artists, one daughter was in such disbelief over what her father had created that she called her husband and asked him to immediately leave work to come and see the show! Celebrating the group's efforts and accomplishments with friends and family not only demonstrates the art therapy program's success but also fosters a sense of community among artists, family members, and others who view the art show. Because older people, and especially those with dementia, are so often isolated and marginalized, bringing forth their vitality, resilience and personality is an important factor in increasing self-esteem and cultivating community.

References

Allen, P. B. (1995). Coyote comes in from the cold: The evolution of the open studio concept. *Art Therapy: Journal of the American Art Therapy Association, 12*(3), 161–166.

Cohen, G. D., Perlstein, S., Chapline, J., Kelly, J., Firth, K. M., & Simmens, S. (2006). The impact of professionally conducted cultural programs on the physical health, mental health, and social functioning of older adults. *The Gerontologist, 46*(6), 726–734.

Flood, M., & Phillips, K. (2007). Creativity in older adults: A plethora of possibilities. [Electronic version]. *Issues in Mental Health Nursing, 28*, 389–411.

Wikström, B. M. (2002). Social interaction associated with visual art discussions: A controlled intervention study. *Aging & Mental Health, 6*(1), 82–87.

Winnicott, D. W. (1971). *Playing and reality.* London: Tavistock Publications.

8 Art Media

Art materials are key tools in an art therapy or creative aging program. The correct tools can unlock a vast potential of expression, learning, and growth. The wrong tools, however, can create frustration, resistance, and even a dangerous experience. This chapter will discuss key considerations for choosing materials, including the appropriateness of the media for the person, situation, and environment; safety considerations, both physical and emotional; developmental considerations; and cultural appropriateness. Art media will be explored alongside the Expressive Therapies Continuum (ETC), along with three revised ETC structures that take into consideration the psychosocial and creative development of older people; cognitive impairment; and multimodal arts. While these new paradigms are not the only alternatives, they offer a way to utilize the power of the ETC to more accurately address the unique needs of some older people.

Tool and Materials

There are endless ways that humans express themselves visually. While common materials such as paint, clay, and pastels are most frequently used in art therapy, anything can become an art material. Found stones can be stacked to create a sculpture, designs can be drawn into dirt with a stick, soap can be intricately patterned on glass with one's fingers. There are so many possibilities for adaptation – with the only limits the interest and ability of the artist, the budget of the program.

In some cases, the art media are used as an extension of ourselves, such as a paintbrush or a pencil. In other cases, hands directly manipulate the material, as with clay. Although for some, a tool can be difficult to control, it keeps hands clean. Others prefer the tactile feeling of working directly with the material. The importance of this distinction is amplified in working with dementia, as well as with people who have arthritis in their hands or other impediments to hand strength or dexterity that make it difficult to grip. If a paintbrush is the most likely tool, the art therapist might need to adapt it to make it easier to grip or give a demonstration on how to use it, perhaps directly holding the older artist's hand and moving with it.

Materials such as clay are typically thought of as kinesthetic, since a person's movement is directly transferred from the hand to the medium. The simplicity of this direct contact can be both grounding and empowering. Using tools such as paint with brushes or palette knives, knitting needles, or pencils allows for more complex and varied manipulation of the medium, but it also requires more advanced skills and focused attention. Aligned developmentally with the perceptual/affective rung of the ETC, tool usage often demands more from the artist and allows for greater freedom. I think about this when informally assessing the need of a person with dementia in my session. Would they benefit from a basic, grounding experience in which they can play and experiment with the medium without negative consequences? Or, would they feel more comfortable distanced from the medium, both physically and emotionally, by using a tool? What adaptations are needed for it to be comfortable and safe? If working directly with the medium, would they prefer wearing gloves so as not to feel the texture directly? If using a paintbrush, would a thinner, thicker, longer, or shorter brush be best? In this way, I am employing the art therapist's third hand, as described in chapter 5, through my assessment and action. It is possible then, to use my third hand to provide a significant amount of assistance and structure so that a person with even advanced dementia might be able to work in the top-rung, cognitive/symbolic/structure. With the loss of abstract thinking that occurs with advanced dementia, significant cognitive and symbolic art expression is severely decreased. However, as the art therapist, I can step in to provide needed support so that some level of expression is possible.

For example, collage can be a very accessible approach to art-making for adolescents who prefer to utilize images that represent themselves and their interests. The multilayered symbolic meaning of collage can be a sophisticated and complex representation of a person. Someone with advanced Alzheimer's disease is unlikely to be able to select images from a magazine that represent what they might create themselves if they were able to. However, if I know the person well enough to know their interests, their color preferences, and so on, I can pre-select and cut images for them to choose from or cut fabric of different textures into a variety of shapes. It is not a perfect solution, as I am making decisions about imagery that may or may not truly be representative, and my hand (and presence) are very much in the artwork, but it does eliminate the steps that they are unable to do, leaving them with a selection of images that can then be arranged purposefully to tell a story about them, with a piece of artwork that can speak for that person on an artistic and symbolic level.

Cognitive Considerations

Certain verbal prompts or media engage the cognitive and symbolic mind and can cause frustration or confusion in people with cognitive challenges such as dementia. An art therapist/teaching artist will move that person to the perceptual/affective or kinesthetic/sensory realm to regain access to their activity and confidence. Art media that primarily utilize the senses of smell and touch are usually the most accessible for those with cognitive impairment. Media that ensure an appealing aesthetic outcome regardless of the artist's abilities are ideal. When choosing media that require abstract thinking, such as decision-making, following directions, or answering questions, for example, structures can be put in place to bridge the gaps of understanding. The art therapist can mediate these barriers by preparing the setting with the art materials ahead of time, and then working side-by-side with the artist to demonstrate use of media or offer support as needed.

Physical Considerations

Hand strength, flexibility, control, visual impairments, hearing, reduced sensory capabilities, limited range of motion, and ambulation are among common reasons for impaired or limited movement. In many cases, traditional art-making tools can be modified or adapted to account for such physical barriers. Accessibility is key. Is the clay difficult to squeeze? Can it be warmed or softened? Is there a better choice than clay? Paint can be watered to make it easier to spread, brushes can be thickened with cloth or paper towels so they are easier to hold. Engaging available senses can help to replace or substitute for an impaired sense (e.g., for loss of vision, engage with music, touch, or smell).

Emotional Considerations

Depression, isolation, and anxiety, among other emotional challenges, can impede or complicate engagement in art-making. For example, it might be helpful to start on the kinesthetic/sensory level to engage a person who has depression with their body. Feeling their body through movement can be grounding, and there is no failure. When it feels safe or the person is more confident, a move up to the perceptual/affective rung can help the person to begin to explore emotions. Isolation might also be addressed by working with partners or with a group on each level of the continuum.

Cultural Considerations

There are numerous considerations for the appropriateness of art-making to ensure it is culturally appropriate. For example, is it assumed that art is for the privileged few to make or observe – those with means and access?

I find that I come up against these expectations/assumptions frequently in my practice. My own bias stems from my formal training in visual art and my personal aesthetic, rooted in Western ideas of beauty – while recognizing that there are others.

Many considerations regarding the safety and functionality of art materials are discussed in this and the previous chapter. And yet, there are many other factors that play out in the ways in which art media carry inherent connotations. It is important to understand how participants think about art. What are the natural ways that arts are already in their lives? What are their aesthetic preferences and experiences with not only formal art materials but alternative arts experiences – for example, sewing, knitting, or weaving? What is their sense of the material, design, style, and craftsmanship? Is art integrated in the very fiber of how they relate to everyday life? It is also imperative to assess and understand our own beliefs about art and culture, asking ourselves the same questions. Do we find the arts to be valued in our particular life or society? By whom and how is it valued?

Quality of Materials

Suggesting that older people should use crayons and play dough can have the effect of diminishing their lives, as if they are capable of using only children's materials. While children's materials are nontoxic and easy to use – two important features for people with dementia or physical challenges – they do not respect the long and rich lives lived by these people. It is possible to use safe, nontoxic materials, but those with more sophisticated and robust qualities are better suited to higher quality artmaking. For example, simple copy paper works fine with crayons but a heavier and higher quality paper designed for drawing, such as bristol, pastel, or watercolor paper has a soft and textured feel that holds the drawing or painting material much better and lasts longer. Better quality paper also feels better to hold in your hand. It can survive aggressive artmaking and layering of media.

The Expressive Therapies Continuum

A helix of creativity, the ETC is a model of creative functioning to classify how people gather and understand information and work with art materials and other forms of expression. Developed by art therapists Kagin and Lusebrink (1978) and expanded by Hinz (2009), the ETC is structured both developmentally and bilaterally for how art media can be used to support and encourage growth in therapy (see Table 8.1 Traditional ETC).

Our brains predominately utilize the left or right hemisphere of the brain depending on the task at hand: Left hemisphere information

Table 8.1 Traditional ETC

Left *"thinking"* brain	Right *"feeling"* brain
FORMAL OPERATIONS STAGE	
Cognitive	**Symbolic**
SCHEMATIC STAGE	
Perceptual	**Affective**
SENSORIMOTOR STAGE	
Kinesthetic	**Sensory**

processing (kinesthetic, perceptual, cognitive) is organized, sequential, linear, verbal, logical, and categorizing. Right hemisphere information processing (sensory, affective, symbolic) is emotional, conceptual, sensory, feeling, intuitive, and spiritual. The ETC explores the way various art media employ the left or right hemisphere. For example, graphite pencils, which require a great deal of motor control and have a deep connection to performing cognitive tasks, draw from the left hemisphere, while paint, which engages a person's feelings, draws more from the right.

The structure of the ETC also parallels Piaget's developmental norms, from the sensorimotor to the schematic to the formal operations stage. For example, a young child explores the world by touching, smelling, and tasting, and thus art media used primarily with sensory skills can support that stage of development. The sensory media can also elicit responses or engagement harking back to a person's early childhood. This can be useful when a client exhibits rigidity in other areas, and tapping into a sensory realm can bypass the overactive thinking brain. Likewise, when a client is lost within their feelings, moving them to a more symbolic or cognitive perspective can be useful to gain reflective distance. Media such as collage and pencil drawing can achieve this.

One underlying assumption of the ETC is that developmental progression is normative in child development; the ETC roughly matches child development from ages 0–15. It is helpful to have this baseline structure, as well as the left and right-brain paradigm from which to enact our therapeutic practice. However, in my work with older people, and especially those with memory loss, this framework in its original form is not as useful as it could be. Therefore, I propose revised versions of the ETC, one for framing work with older people and another for those with dementia.

ETC for Older People

The developmental evolution of the adult is more nuanced than the dramatic changes that happen in childhood. However, these developmental stages are no less important and should be a primary consideration when working with adults and older adults. They include psychosocial adjustments from self-centeredness to a more generative and external view of the self and the world; a focus on looking back, giving back, and leaving a legacy; and a greater capacity to solve complex problems, utilizing a more diverse set of skills than their younger counterparts.

In adapting the traditional ETC, it is important to know the challenges or barriers that are present for older people and to help them to find new ways to bridge or circumvent them using their strengths, experiences, skills, and the things they still can do.

As discussed in chapter 3, new links between creativity and wisdom have been identified, as well as the older mind's tremendous capacity for adaptive, creative thinking. We know that as a person ages, they develop a greater need for self-expression. Through their mastery and integration of life experience, many older adults feel an increased capacity for creativity. And we know that creative expression can foster confidence, inspiration, motivation, and insight (Stephenson, 2014). Thus, reconceptualizing the powerful ETC model alongside a blended concept of the developmental stages of older adults as outlined by Erikson (1959), Erikson and Erikson (1997), Tornstam (2005), Stowe and Cooney (2015), and Diehl and Wahl (2020) is a more appropriate representation for our purposes.

Identity, Connection, and Motivation

The traditional ETC grounds each level in Piaget's developmental hierarchy. The ETC for older people pairs Paiget's stages of child cognitive development with developmental and functional capabilities that are relevant to an older person in their cognitive, physical, and emotional functioning. It is often a loss in these areas that impedes well-being: physical health, cognitive performance, physical functioning, the sense of personal control and mastery, social skills, and a sense of personal and existential integrity.

The goals of the ETC, as revised for the developmental uniqueness of the older person, are hierarchically aligned parallel to Piaget's stages that ground the traditional ETC (See Table 8.2. ETC for Older People).

Corresponding to the bottom rung of sensory motor in the traditional ETC, the ETC for older people is motivation. As noted in chapter six, fostering the motivation to persevere can help a person cope with a decline in motor and sensory functioning. We saw this reflected in Marcia's continuation of art making despite suffering from chronic fatigue syndrome, or Marina diligently attending the open studio despite experiencing debilitating arthritis pain.

The middle rung, aligned with the schematic stages of Piaget, is connection. At this level, feeling states may be broader, a person may feel

Table 8.2 ETC for Older People

Left "thinking" brain	*Right "feeling" brain*
IDENTITY/LEGACY	
(Formal Operations Stage)	
Cognitive	**Symbolic**
Advanced capacity to understand and utilize cognitive and symbolic thinking to solve complex problems	
CONNECTION	
(Schematic Stage)	
Perceptual	**Affective**
Feeling states may be broader, connected across generations, higher capacity for empathy	
MOTIVATION	
(Sensorimotor Stage)	
Kinesthetic	**Sensory**
Decline in fine motor and sensory abilities	

connected across generations, and may experience a higher capacity for empathy. This feature of connection is notable in most of the stories presented in this book–connection is vital for maintaining health and well-being, and staving off isolation and loneliness.

And the highest level, or formal operations, is identity and legacy. With a refined capacity to understand and utilize cognitive and symbolic thinking to solve complex problems, art-making at this level can be utilized for deep reflection. The cognition and symbolic expression employed by Adeena exemplifies the expansive potential of how a person can explore their identity and legacy through art making.

Knowing how various media/activities elicit certain types of expression and bridge potential barriers, art therapists can use the ETC to engage older adults along this continuum. In recognizing that certain verbal prompts or media engage the cognitive or symbolic mind and can cause frustration or confusion in a person coping with dementia, an art therapist can move that person to the perceptual/affective or kinesthetic/sensory realm, where they regain access to greater self-expression and confidence.

Bilateral Adjustments in the Aging Brain

Bilateral brain functioning is more integrated in older people because of life experience using both sides of the brain to solve problems. Older brains utilize their capacity more efficiently. The ETC for older people therefore places less emphasis on the left/right brain dichotomy. Dr. Gene Cohen noted (2005) that, as people age, activities that had once been left- or right-brain dominant draw more from bilateral integration of the left and right brain hemispheres; this occurs especially for tasks such as short-term memory, word-finding, and facial recognition. The hemispheric asymmetry reduction in older adults (HAROLD) model (Cabeza, 2002) indicates that the aging brain compensates for neural decline by re-organizing and changing brain hemisphere connectivity. According to the HAROLD model, older people's brains utilize hemispheres more bilat-erally than those of younger people (Cabeza et al., 2002) in studies of memory retrieval, working memory, perception, and inhibitory control (Cabeza, 2002). Hemispheric reorganization changes occur to compen-sate for decline in naming and word retrieval (Höller-Wallscheid et al., 2017; Hoyau et al., 2017).

Thus, while the ETC was developed as a bilateral concept, it is possible that the distinction between the functions of the left and right brain hemispheres is less pronounced in older people. In fact, observing art-making processes with older people could potentially yield a valuable contribution to our knowledge of hemispheric brain functioning and adaptation in old age. Adnan et al. (2019) found that greater integration of brain regions in older adults, is positively associated with more creativity.

Rose, introduced in chapter 2, is an example of how the integration of left and right brain functioning and drawing on all three steps in the continuum ladder resulted in self-affirming, satisfying creativity.

Rose explained how her approach to making art has changed as she has gotten older. While she had more confidence, she felt that physical limitations, such as arthritis, at times prevented her from doing what she wanted to do. For example, she said that her arthritis didn't affect holding the paintbrush, but changed the way she moved it. After shoulder surgery, she began drawing and painting with her left, non-dominant hand because her right arm was immobilized. As a result, her work be-came completely abstract. She noted how she felt liberated by this change, while at the same time empowered by the fact that she could continue to work without the use of her right hand. Subsequently, Rose used playful stories to guide her work. Figure 2.3 *Racing Colors* is a pastel drawing depicting a story she invented about the primary colors (red, yellow, and blue) running across the page, when suddenly black enters the picture and chases the colors back to the other side. Using a story to guide and structure her work emerged as a new and creative approach that motivated her to continue her engagement in and enjoyment of making art. She expressed great joy in her ability to continue making art despite the immobilization of her dominant arm and, in particular, felt empowered.

The Revised ETC for Older People

Below is an elaboration on the revised ETC stages for older people. As noted above, the revised older adult development stage is paired with the traditional Piaget child development stage, beginning with the earliest developmental stage that appears on the bottom rung.

Motivation/Sensorimotor

Motivation may be derived from one's thinking brain and cognitive decision-making. However, the visceral components of sensory and kinesthetic media often draw a person's attention and action, bypassing higher cognitive functioning. The ease of using this type of media, their accessibility, and the low level of commitment required lend themselves to baseline or introductory engagement in art-making. People who might not be interested in or intimidated by art-making, those who are creatively stuck, and those with cognitive or physical challenges are most likely to be drawn in at this level.

Connection/Schematic

At the schematic level, there is planning and connection to thinking/feeling/action. Here, the need to be connected, the ability to use art-making to connect with other people, happens in a more purposeful way, in which the individual has greater awareness of their visibility and presence among others. The artwork and/or process of creating art is a catalyst to bring people together, to engage in an activity side by side, to influence one another, to share work, and to engage in conversation.

Identity and Legacy/Formal Operations

Formal thought (postformal, for adults) is the stage of conscious, abstract thinking and planning. For many older people who are not experiencing dementia, this level corresponds developmentally with legacy and identity development. Contemplating one's future and past, considering what they might leave behind for the world, reconciling who they are, are all features that demand a high level of cognition. Art media that can convey complex, symbolic meaning and require a higher level of executive functioning fall into this category. For those who have dementia, the art therapist can step in as needed as the cognitive planner to create structure and some guidance.

Adeena, introduced in chapter 2, focused her work on paying homage to others, and her work exemplifies the Identity & Legacy rung. Her pieces often included discarded or found objects that she turned into artwork. She created an interactive art piece in which people could take little pods with poetry written on them.

This top level is the one that can be best aligned with adult developmental theory, and also the level that can be inaccessible to those with dementia. The therapist must be aware of limitations in the older artist with respect to 1) their ability for self-reflection, 2) executive functioning, and 3) capacity for broad creative expression. For those without dementia, there is tremendous possibility to utilize this level of formal/postformal thought, drawing on wisdom, experience, life review, and self-reflection to explore one's identity and legacy.

For *Love and War* (Figure 8.1 Love and War) Adeena collected honey locust seed pods that had fallen to the ground and covered them in rice paper on which she wrote English war poems and 17th-century Japanese love poems written by women to their lovers. Some pods were hung for display, while others were placed in a bowl for people to take with them. She hoped the interactive nature of the poetry pods would ignite further communication with the exhibition-goers, intrigued by the "implication or promise of further interaction." Adeena described how making art about others was based on deep respect for the person, transforming them and giving them a new life in a way. She said, "I have empathy for someone who's achieved something that's not monumental yet very important in ways that younger people couldn't even imagine. I am respecting them and respecting myself at the same time." Adeena's artistic

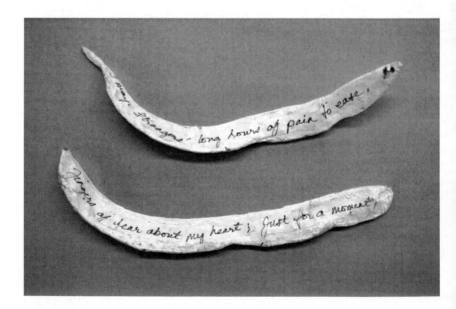

Figure 8.1 Love and War.

expression using this nontraditional medium drew deeply upon the meaning of her own life and the lives of others, exemplifying the complex and layered meaning possible in postformal thought.

Another example of the legacy/formal operations stage can be seen in how the relationship between Elena and Rosa developed through participation in the open art studio and their acknowledgment of their friendship in the art itself. Elena and Rose became friends in the open studio art group. Although they lived in the same cooperative apartment complex, they had never met. Both women were among the younger participants and were born and raised in Puerto Rico. Both were skilled artists who demonstrated confidence working in a variety of media, in styles ranging from abstraction to realism. Often they could be observed sitting at the table drawing portraits of each other. This intrigued other artists, who began to engage in the same activity. Making a portrait is difficult; it is an intimate experience for both parties. The artist closely observing the fine details of a person for extended lengths of time can feel invasive or uncomfortable to some subjects. And yet, this deep visual exploration was not only accepted, it was embraced time and time again. Through the years, the portraits recorded who was present. Details were also honest and authentic, without a wrinkle or gray hair altered. The portraits evidence a high level of connection, comfort, and acceptance among the group participants and reflect people witnessing one another in the most direct possible way in visual art.

The Revised ETC for Dementia

The initial assessments I make with people with dementia concern safety and capability. What resources does the person have access to? What are some barriers and/or challenges? Access might include interest or experience in art-making, or mobility. Challenges might be poor vision, restricted mobility, or significant cognitive decline. Thus, my interventions are led by the presenting opportunity. If a person has arthritis in their hands, which makes it difficult to hold small items such as pastels or control a tool such as a pencil, the media chosen will be one that they can utilize easily, maybe clay or paint. If they have advanced memory loss, it would be unfair to ask them to engage in thematic art-making or projects that require abstract thinking or imagination. Rather, the art-making will be more sensory/ kinesthetic or affective, where there is a great deal of freedom of expression without limiting factors such as expectation for realism or story formation.

I find it helpful to think of these considerations alongside the ETC, as it helps to make obvious the abilities, limitations, opportunities, and challenges before me with each client. At the same time, a revised ETC appropriate for developmental and functional factors in older people with dementia is useful not only in case planning but also in training students, therapists, and teaching artists (see Table 8.3 ETC for Dementia).

Table 8.3 ETC for Dementia

Left "thinking" brain	Right "feeling" brain
STRUCTURE	
(Formal Operations Stage)	
Cognitive	**Symbolic**
This level is limited as dementia advances and capacity for abstract thinking diminishes. Can be used to provide structure in which the perceptual and/or affective can exist more freely.	
FREEDOM	
(Schematic Stage)	
Perceptual	**Affective**
For those with dementia, this might be the highest level achieved in the ETC hierarchy, due to the abstract thinking required in the top level. This level can be very effective at providing an outlet for emotions that cannot be adequately expressed verbally.	
GROUNDING	
(Sensorimotor Stage)	
Kinesthetic	**Sensory**
There can be some challenges with overlap between art materials and other sensory items. Confusion increases as dementia advances, but kinesthetic and sensory remain the most accessible realms for artistic engagement.	

The ETC for dementia has three layers – grounding (sensorimotor), freedom (the schematic stage), and structure (formal operations).

Grounding

There can be some challenges with overlap between art materials and other sensory items, such as food. A person with dementia might confuse art materials for food. While confusion increases as dementia advances, the body-oriented kinesthetic and sensory realms are the most accessible realms for artistic engagement as they can be experienced immediately and directly between the body and the medium, grounding a person on the here and now. Engaging in sensory movement is a safe, easy, fun, successful beginning to introducing more art-making that involves tools, conceptualization, and greater complexity.

Magda, a Polish-speaking woman with advanced dementia, demonstrated her adeptness at manipulating Model Magic. Typically, it is a material designed for children and can have an infantilizing effect on adults. However, it is nontoxic, clean, very pliable, paintable, and at the moment, for Magda, in the hospital unit, it was the best choice. Magda had arthritis and had difficulty working in other media such as collage and painting. But, the tactile and accessible qualities of Model Magic enticed her. Magda and I were not able to communicate verbally because of our language differences. I observed her to be friendly but distant from her peers, and I was unsure if this was because others could not speak Polish or that dementia rendered verbal communication difficult in general. Her demeanor changed, though, as she molded the Model Magic, crafting a half dozen small clay pierogis. Delighted by her creation, she smiled and spoke to the group, her peers, replying to their appreciation of her work. Modeling the clay seemed to be grounding in that her hands recreated that which was familiar in an unfamiliar, or at least disconnected, environment.

Freedom

Ideally everyone will experience freedom to express themselves. As an art therapist, I do all I can to remove barriers preventing this freedom. Barriers might be emotional such as fear of exposure or fear of failure; they can be physical such as restricted mobility or low vision, or organic such as functional decline in the brain due to dementia. Often, imposing some sort of structure can give room for freedom to occur. This concept is discussed in greater depth in chapter 9. Rena exemplifies how such structure can yield to a freedom of expression for a person who was legally blind and had Alzheimer's disease. Rena was very interested in circles, as she could understand their shape and they gave her a framework to connect with art-making. She frequently exclaimed the word "circles" aloud, which enhanced the connection of Rena with her circles. As a blind woman, Rena relied heavily on her sense of touch, although she was able to see high contrast, well-lit colors. In nearly all of our interactions with her, we gave her some sort of a circle to work within. For those with dementia, this might be the highest level achieved in the ETC hierarchy, due to the abstract thinking required in the top level. And yet, this level can be very effective at providing an outlet for emotions that cannot be adequately expressed verbally. Feelings are still very much present in the person with dementia, but they need new avenues to express them.

At times, for Rena, the avenue was a piece of heavy watercolor with a thick circle drawn in the center, usually black, purple, or red, with a permanent or magic marker, or an oil pastel. Sometimes, the circle was a piece of textured paper cut in the shape of a circle and then glued to a piece of paper. Other times, the cut circle paper was of a highly contrasting color – for example, a black circle on white paper. Yet another approach was to create a circle on paper using twisted tissue paper, twine, or other materials that made it tactically obvious. Once the circle was created (by someone else), Rena felt free to draw, paint, or collage within, outside, and across the circle. The circle gave her a sensory, visual, and conceptual structure that guided her work, and most importantly, allowed her to have freedom to play. While this preparation work can very much be considered the work of the third hand, it can also be viewed as formal operations work, aligning with the top level of the ETC. With Rena, the art therapists utilized formal operations to create a structured art-making environment, so that she would be free to express herself in the affective/symbolic realm and, at times, the sensory/kinesthetic. Because of Rena's cognitive loss due to Alzheimer's disease, she no longer had access to abstract thinking, thematic or structural planning, or other forms of executive functioning. Because the therapists were able to take over these realms and give her the structure and ability to engage in the art-making, the art therapy proved beneficial to her.

Structure

Structure, introduced in the section above, can also be constructed by the artists themselves. In this way, following a reliable procedure or pursuing a familiar theme creates a supportive environment within which a person is able to explore art expression. My observation of Wayne's work made me curious about how his familiar imagery might have allowed for increased experimentation with art making.

Wayne experienced rapid-onset memory loss that completely transformed his independence. It was unclear what had caused the decline, and unfortunately, during my time working with him, it did not improve. Nevertheless, Wayne attended many art therapy sessions where he painted a familiar theme again and again. He depicted two men in many of his works; sometimes they were standing side by side, each next to a tree, or reclining on a bed, each in a small room adjacent to one another. This structure component, however, can be limited as dementia becomes more advanced and the capacity for abstract thinking diminishes. The art therapist can use this, however, to provide structure, prompting, or a framework within which the perceptual and/or affective can exist more freely/comfortably. However, for some, symbolic elements emerge without much structure needed.

Wayne's depiction of the two men resembled the drawing of a young child with X-ray features such as the skeleton showing. They were without clothing, with the exception of a colorful strand hanging down across the chest of each, resembling a necktie or an enlarged heart. The expression on the men was that of contentment. Wayne titled one of these paintings *Two Men Born at the Same Time (Not Brothers)*. This title confused me. However, upon learning that his life's work was in Buddhist studies, and observing his visits with a friend who was dressed in a suit and tie, it seemed possible that the paintings symbolized their friendship, or perhaps incorporated his Buddhist worldview. The symbolic elements of Wayne's painting communicated far more about his life than he was able to express verbally.

Multimedia ETC for Dementia

A group of 12 older women with mild to moderate dementia gathered weekly for a dance/movement and art therapy group. Beginning first with seated stretching and moving to music, participants were encouraged to follow the leader with small and large range of motion movements, followed by independent motions in response to music and others present. From the movement circle, participants made a quick transition to a table with art materials prearranged. Participants were then encouraged to represent their favorite movement from the previous exercise, at first by making a gesture with a paintbrush in their hand. This was followed by connecting that movement to a color or colors. From there, participants used water colors to reenact their favorite movements in color, shape, and line. The energy at the beginning of the art-making portion of the group was higher than what is typical in an art group that begins without the movement preamble. After a short time painting, participants settled into their process, quieting their bodies as evidenced by smaller, more focused brushstrokes and increased intentionality in the painting, as well as a decrease in talking among participants.

Incorporating multiple modes of expression can foster a deeper experience, in which the body and senses are connected more purposefully (see Table 8.4 Multimedia ETC for Dementia).

Table 8.4 Multimedia ETC for Dementia

Left "thinking" brain	*Right "feeling" brain*
STRUCTURE	
Cognitive	**Symbolic**
Art: Draw a house/face	Art: Collage representing self
Music: Compose a rhythm	Music: Compose a song
Movement: Create a new dance	Movement: Develop a character with scarves
FREEDOM	
Perceptual	**Affective**
Art: Draw with oil pastel	Art: Paint with watercolors
Music: Sing song from childhood	Music: Words, tone that express a feeling
Movement: Pass string, share a thought	Movement: Move body, express a feeling
GROUNDING	
Kinesthetic	**Sensory**
Art: Explore clay	Art: Smell spices and citrus
Music: Tap rhythm on table or body	Music: Hum, feel vibrations in chest
Movement: Big arm stretches	Movement: Rub hand together, warmth & sound

Applying the ETC to work with people who have dementia, it makes good sense to envision how various modalities might be situated on the ETC ladder. As described above, enlivening the senses prior to or as part of making visual art can lead to a more sustained and rewarding experience. Likewise, moving from one artistic modality to another can be beneficial. For example, one possibility is for music or movement to first ground the person in their body in the sensory/kinesthetic/grounding realm, with the visual art then pulling for action on the perceptual/affective/freedom level. The grounding kinesthetic dance/movement component can allow for a quicker transition to art-making, deeper engagement in the artwork, and improved facilitation of perceptual and affective expression.

Concluding Thoughts

The traditional ETC is an excellent framework on which to build. The concepts presented in this chapter are new and, at this point, theoretical, with only limited application to test their viability. It would be beneficial for these ideas to be explored, assessed, and revised as needed so they can evolve into the most useful framework possible. My hope is that you, the reader, will be inspired to stretch the ETC and its application into more nuanced territory.

References

Adnan, A., Beaty, R., Silvia, P., Spreng, R. N., & Turner, G. R. (2019). Creative aging: Functional brain networks associated with divergent thinking in older and younger adults. *Neurobiology of Aging*, *75*, 150–158. https://doi.org/10.1016/j.neurobiolaging.2018.11.004

Cabeza, R. (2002). Hemispheric asymmetry reduction in older adults: The HAROLD model. *Psychology and Aging*, *17*(1), 85–100. https://doi-org.ezproxyles.flo.org/10.1037/0882–7974.17.1.85

Cabeza, R., Anderson, N. D., Locantore, J. K., & McIntosh, A. R. (2002). Aging gracefully: Compensatory brain activity in high-performing older adults. *Neuroimage*, *17*(3), 1394–1402. https://doi-org.ezproxyles.flo.org/10.1006/nimg.2002.1280

Cohen, G. D. (2005). *The mature mind: The positive power of the aging brain*. New York: Basic Books.

Diehl, M., & Wahl, H.-W. (2020). Risks and potentials of adult development and aging: Understanding the challenges and opportunities of successful aging. In *The psychology of later life: A contextual perspective* (pp. 153–180). American Psychological Association. https://doi-org.ezproxyles.flo.org/10.1037/0000185–007

Erikson, E. H. (1959). *Identity and the life cycle*. New York: Norton

Erikson, E. H., & Erikson, J. M. (1997). *The life cycle completed: Extended version with new chapters on the Ninth Stage of development*. New York: W.W. Norton & Company, Inc.

Hinz, L. D. (2009). *Expressive therapies continuum: A framework for using art in therapy*. Hove, GBR: Psychology Press.

Höller-Wallscheid, M. S., Thier, P., Pomper Jörn, K., & Lindner A. (2017). Bilateral recruitment of prefrontal cortex in working memory is associated with task demand but not with age. *Proceedings of the National Academy of Sciences of the United States of America*, *114*(5), E830.

Hoyau, E., Boudiaf, N., Cousin, E., Pichat, C., Fournet N., Krainik, A., Jaillard, A., & Baciu, M. (2017). Aging modulates the hemispheric specialization during word production. *Frontiers in Aging Neuroscience*, *9*(125). doi:10.3389/fnagi. 2017.00125. https://www.frontiersin.org/articles/10.3389/fnagi.2017.00125/full

Kagin, S., & Lusebrink, V. (1978). The expressive therapies continuum. *Art Psychotherapy*, *5*, 171–180.

Stephenson, R. C. (2014). Art in aging: How identity as an artist can transcend the challenges of aging. *International Journal of Creativity and Human Development*, *1*(3). https://www.creativityjournal.net/component/k2/item/244-art-in-aging-how-identity-as-an-artist-can-transcend-the-challenges-of-aging

Stowe, J. D., & Cooney, T. M. (2015). Examining Rowe and Kahn's concept of successful aging: Importance of taking a life course perspective. *Gerontologist*, *55*(1), 43–50. doi:10.1093/geront/gnu055

Tornstam, L. (2005). *Gerotranscendence: A developmental theory of positive aging*. New York: Springer Publishing Company.

9 Art and Dementia

"Too much muchness." – Rhonda

Robert sat quietly in his wheelchair, his gaze soft and not directed at anything in particular. He was not interested in participating in art therapy or any other group activity. Although we encouraged him, he remained mostly asleep in his chair. One day, I stayed at the program longer than usual, overlapping with the time a musician played piano for the group. I couldn't believe my eyes when I saw Robert stand up from his wheelchair and dance in the center of the circle of chairs, singing the words of a song he knew. It was as if a switch had been turned on. Suddenly he was animated, energetic, and had a seemingly different personality.

Like music, visual art and movement can be very effective in dementia work. While a person is not able to execute a thematic painting or drawing, the visceral qualities of the materials often invoke an emotional response, with the individual expressing frustration, anger, contentment, or joy through paint strokes, taking risks as they participate in the creative process. Because of encouragement from others and the safe environment of the art room, older adults with dementia are able to remain motivated to engage with the art materials, even though they might be disoriented.

Dementia is likely the most common presenting illness that arts therapists and teaching artists are confronted with in their practice with older people. Working from a person-centered lens, the importance of reclaiming communication is the overarching paradigm. This chapter builds on the goals identified in chapter 6, and the structure and process outlined in chapter 7, adjusting and applying them to align with the needs of those with dementia.

Beyond Words

Creative arts therapists and teaching artists working with people who have Alzheimer's disease and other forms of dementia explore tools and techniques that can be adapted to those who struggle with loss of memory and restricted ability to communicate. While techniques to increase mastery of artistic expression can be taught, the focus is mostly on fostering a sense of purpose, social connectivity, and self-esteem – factors that are essential to the health and well-being of all older people. Although it is difficult to measure these types of improvements, they are noticed at times in the subtle ways a person expands their range of expression, takes greater risks in their artwork, or develops social connections with others in the group.

Using art therapy with people who have dementia can have a lasting, positive impact on mental alertness and increased sociability (Rusted et al., 2006) and improved cognitive function (Lee et al., 2019; Zhao et al., 2019). Improvements have been observed in the quality of life (Hattori et al., 2011). In particular, art therapy for Alzheimer's disease enhances attention, interest, emotion, and mood. With dementia, it has been shown to reduce stress-related behaviors (Mimica & Dubravka, 2011). Studies carried out with persons with aphasia involved in continuing art therapy demonstrate the growth of nonverbal communication (Horovitz, 2005; Sacchett et al., 1999). Sacchett et al. (1999) found that drawing increased the ability of participants to understand, name, and gesture when practiced and developed in structured therapy. Likewise, art therapy has contributed to improving attention, physical coordination, visual-spatial processing, and language recovery with people recovering from stroke (Kim et al., 2008). Gonen and Soroker (2000) found that art therapy helps patients address feelings about stroke and loss of function, as well as motivation and self-expression, while Symons et al. (2011) identified the social benefits of art therapy participation.

Dementia, encompassing a range of conditions and diseases in which there is deterioration in memory, thinking, behavior, and the ability to perform everyday activities, is one of the major causes of disability and dependency for older people. Dementia has a significant physical, psychological, social, and economic impact not only on the diagnosed individual, but also on caregivers, families, and society. Where there is no cure for the underlying cause of some forms of dementia (e.g., Alzheimer's disease), there are ways to improve the quality of life of affected individuals. It is an accepted opinion that treatment of dementia should aim to enhance quality of life and improve mood and behavior (American Psychiatric Association, 2011). No doubt, Alzheimer's disease and other dementias are heartbreaking for both those experiencing them and their families. Loss of memory, and ultimately the basic means of self-care and functioning, devastate a person's ability to maintain their independence and severely impact their quality of life. But dementia does not remove a life lived and all that has been experienced; though the mechanism for expressing it is blocked, the internal life of that person is not extinguished. The arts can be a window through which a person in this situation can express themselves nonverbally. It takes time and effort to help unlock the new portal, but it is possible, and remarkable things transpire.

It is important to recognize and acknowledge the loss and pain and to be aware of the many facets of that person's life that have changed, not to mention the effect on family and caregivers. One part of the therapeutic encounter is to provide support to and understanding of that person as they grieve their former selves and adjust to an increasingly confusing, disjointed, and unrecognizable life. Another part, though, is to support the strengths that remain. I am aware that I cannot help a person to regain their memory, reverse progressive disease, or bring back the many losses they have experienced. But what I can do is to honor and value the person who is in front of me, regardless of however much time they have left to live. So, rather than attempting to make very small and very unlikely improvements in memory for a split second, I choose to connect with that person, with who they are now, and help them to experience comfort, connection and joy.

Therapeutic Goals

The same goals presented in chapter 6 – artist identity, connection, and motivation – are relevant in work with dementia. However, they are achieved through adjusted approaches and with a shift in expectations about outcomes. (The text in parenthesis is a companion goal that might be in better alignment with the needs or abilities of the artist with dementia.)

Artist Identity (Visual Communication)

Communication is a basic human need. When a person loses the ability to process language and words become an impossible tool for communication, that person is at greater risk for decreased health and well-being. Research shows that psychosocial treatment of dementia improves cognition, quality of life for patient and family caregivers, and the reduction of neuropsychiatric symptoms (Dugmore et al., 2015; Teri et al., 2005; Logsdon & Teri, 2018), helping patients to "becom[e] a person again" (Hunter et al., 2016). The creative arts therapies can be especially beneficial to an older person with dementia. This expressive psychosocial approach can improve self-esteem and promote a sense of belonging through embodied communication that fosters the kind of meaningful engagement Kontos and Grigorovich (2018a, 2018b) describe as central to effective person-centered care. One of the powerful aspects of creative arts therapy is that, for people who struggle with the spoken word, working with the arts as a communication tool can be incredibly liberating, relieving the stress and anxiety that talking may create (Stephenson, 2015). An alternative means to communicate relieves the burden of language impairment (Abraham, 2005; Schall et al., 2015) and reduces stress-related behaviors

(Mimica & Dubravka, 2011). Zaidel's (2013) research shows that the communicative nature of art is neuronally more damage resistant than language, and communication through art can have a lasting, positive impact on mental alertness, increased sociability, and improved physical and social engagement.

Connecting with those who have dementia through their expressions in art, along with small, nuanced forms of nonverbal or limited verbal communication, we are able to find new ways to unlock doors of communication that have been shut and even create new avenues. As our clients become increasingly isolated due to dementia, it is of utmost importance that through their art-making and reflection upon their artwork, their peers' work, the therapist's presence, support, and guidance throughout, we foster a sense of community.

Lila

Lila, a 90-year-old woman with arthritis and advanced Alzheimer's disease, was no longer able to speak English and instead spoke only a few words in Russian, her first language. With the loss of memory, language, and, as a result, relationship, she had become isolated. In art therapy, she was unable to paint conceptual imagery because she had lost the ability to think abstractly. If we had given Lila a set of instructions, she couldn't have followed them. Instructions dictate so much of our life. To a person with significant memory loss, who cannot understand instructions, how confusing the world must seem.

Lost in a world where she could no longer understand phrases, Lila became excited and focused when art materials were put before her. Painting for Lila was a multi-sensory experience in which she held and used paintbrushes in both her hands or, at times, enjoyed the sensation of paint on her fingers as she massaged it onto the soft, textured watercolor paper. Lila's eyes twinkled with pride as her painting emerged, reveling in the colors that reflected back and the recognition she earned from friends and caregivers, such as in *Sunflower* (See Figure 9.1 Sunflower). Painting with a brush in each hand, the synchronous moments of her arms turned the painting into a form of dance as well. Other times, her fingers tiptoed across the painting, leaving her fingerprints in the paint marking her process. Witnessing her making art demonstrated to me how she was developing alternative paths of expression through visual art. Lila's visceral response to the art media enlivened her, and I felt her joy as I watched her eyes pay close attention to the paint on her fingertips, open wider to the evolving colors appearing on the paper, and then connect intently with my eyes, as if looking for confirmation or approval. The painting process was a vessel through which Lila was able to connect with her world. Years later, when I look at this painting, I remember clearly her painting it, her bright eyes and nimble fingers in movement. I felt joy

Figure 9.1 Sunflower.

being in her presence as she painted it, and that feeling has stayed with me to this day.

Time and time again, I have noticed how even those with advanced Alzheimer's disease can improve self-expression, communication, and connection to others.

Rhonda

Rhonda was a keen observer of those around her, and her work was intuitively reflective of her environment. She noticed what others were doing and the colors and shapes they were using. When others were laughing, she quietly studied them. She painted with a concentration that equaled that of her observation, carefully mixing colors, often creating a diverse palette of cool blues and greens. Rhonda was easily distracted into observing others, no doubt a product of her long career as a child psychologist. A gentle, inquisitive 85-year-old, Rhonda was eager to paint when the materials were laid out for her. Her facial expressions became more fluid as she began to drag her brush across the thick watercolor paper, perhaps reacting to the vibrant color that appeared or the feel of the brush in her hand moving across the page.

Rhonda often paused to examine the artwork others in the group were making. When her neighbor used red, that same color often appeared in Rhonda's painting. When an artist across the table blended blue and red together, Rhonda often copied that as well. Her work had its own recognizable style, but it was influenced by that of her peers. While she had great difficulty expressing herself verbally, struggling for minutes to release a word or two, she communicated much more fluidly through her paintings. And yet, her words, when she found them, could be profound. One day, upon viewing her artwork, she exclaimed, "Too much muchness." Unlike most of her paintings that are subdued, with blues and greens, this particular painting filled much of the canvas with many colors that blended together, including reds, yellows, and oranges, painted on top of a magazine cut out that was pre-pasted onto the paper. Her critique, "too much muchness," captured the work perfectly. For Rhonda, her artwork stood as a marker of that day – a visual note giving evidence that she was there, a group member who not only expressed herself but made a connection with the expression of others.

Connection (Reduce Social Isolation)

Individuals with dementia struggle to achieve connection and are at high risk for compounding medical and emotional problems due to loneliness and social isolation.

Making art together in a group allows them to communicate without words. Participants are able to maintain their connection to this small community through the art-making process. While many of the participants attended the program when they were no longer welcome at any others due to the advanced stages of the illness, these men and women continued to express a great need to communicate with others.

Making art together in a group allows people to communicate without words. Mostly led by the group leaders, the intent was to make bridges of connection between the artists. Through this intentional movement from individual to group, artists could visually see how they were essential members of a group.

The focus of the NYU CATS art therapy program at the Lenox Hill Neighborhood House CARE Program, attended by Elena, was designed for those with Alzheimer's disease to provide a community setting where people could socialize with peers, in addition to providing respite for caregivers. What was most important was that people felt they belonged there, that it was their community. Thus, while the artwork of the individual was valued, it was also a point of visual connection between group members and by the artists with themselves. Family members and caregivers reported marked changes in behavior of several participants upon returning home from the program. For example, Joe was reportedly argumentative with his wife and at times combative, visibly unhappy, and angry. However, while in our presence, he was usually smiling, cracking jokes, and seeking the friendship of others in the room. We surmised that, in part, Joe's improved behavior was due to the safe, supportive, person-centered environment, where a person with memory impairment "fits in." While many of the participants attended the program when they were no longer welcome at any others, due to the advanced stages of the illness, these men and women continued to express a great need to communicate with others. Despite having lost the ability to speak, they shared their thoughts and feelings through art media. It was an incredible opportunity to get to know these people through their expressions in art, along with small, nuanced forms of nonverbal or limited verbal communication, and to find new ways to unlock doors of communication that had been shut, or even to create new avenues using artistic expression.

For example, in a group art-making session, each participant made a drawing on a precut piece of paper. These were later assembled with the others to create a community artwork that reflected the contributions of each artist. This two-part process drew from the strengths of the artists. It could be overwhelming to participate outright in group art-making, since group work requires collaboration, communication, and flexibility. Additionally, a process that would require participants to move, reach, or see details across the table or the room could be challenging. In this process, each person began at their own pace, making their own piece. Group leaders devised a plan for how the individual pieces would be assembled. Sometimes we would create a pre-existing frame for the final piece, or the precut pieces would fit together like a puzzle when reassembled, such as in *Group Collage* (Figure 9.2 Group Collage). Other times, the format was more fluid, and display of the artwork would be decided among the group. Through this intentional movement from individual to group, artists could visually see how they were essential members of a group. In these sessions, the discussion of the art focused on the final piece rather than specifics of individual work. Some participants lost sight of their own work or couldn't remember that they made it, but none-theless, they were interested in the piece before them and were eager to comment on it: "It's a masterpiece!" "Let's sell it for one million dollars!"

There are multiple ways that connection can be fostered and supported through arts engagement. Four components that are evident in any art therapy or creative aging session are:

1. Taking a risk in the presence of others
2. Sharing and discussing artwork
3. Facilitation by leaders of connections among members
4. Participants connecting to themselves through artistic discovery

The first two are naturally occurring, assuming the session has at least two people in it (a therapist and one client, for example) and that there is time for reflection and discussion.

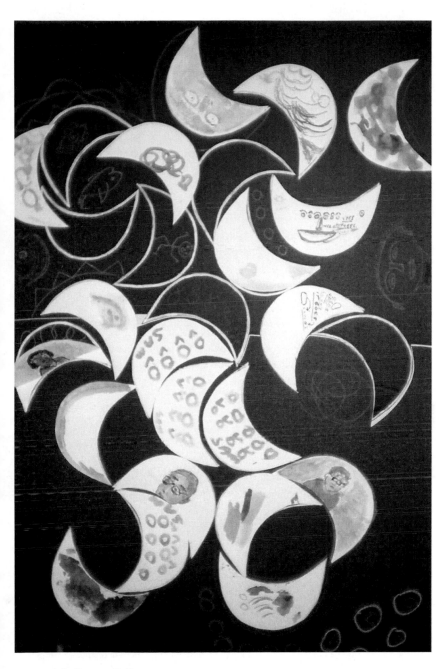

Figure 9.2 Group Collage.

The art therapist or teaching artist might be called upon to help participants work together or to notice or acknowledge one another in some instances. In a group art therapy session with people who had advanced Alzheimer's disease and who were withdrawn, we facilitated a visual/ physical activity that literally connected the participants to one another. With a large ball of red yarn, participants were asked to pass the ball to another member seated around the rectangular table and to greet that person as they transferred the yarn. The purposeful action of passing the yarn to another, with the visual record as the yarn unspooled, allowed people to form literal connections with one another. Where there had been 12 individuals quietly sitting alone with themselves, the activity enlivened the mood and energy level. The final visual product was a complex pattern of red yarn, pathed across the table in all directions. We mounted the work on a board using glue and displayed it on the wall, concrete evidence that each participant was connected to that community. While the connection fades once participants leave, what remains for each person is the imprint of that belonging and connection.

Motivation (Joy)

Joy is not often a therapeutic goal. Therapeutic goals are usually behaviors that can be measured as markers of mental health improvement. Some might question how we might ascertain efficacy from observing certain behaviors in a dementia arts program, such as increased smiling, eye contact with others, a more erect or forward body position, and so on. These markers are all valid indicators of positive engagement. But what is the purpose of positive engagement? I would argue that the benchmark for a "successful" arts encounter is not unlike the one we all use in our lives. We are more likely to seek a "joyful life" rather than a "positively engaged life." Thus, in my work with older people, including those with dementia, I aim to foster joy.

Motivation can propel a person to accomplish something. It also emerges from feeling of enjoyment and the desire to get more of it. Thus, by igniting joy through art-making, motivation to further engage expands. And as noted above, more engagement can lead to improved connection and communication. Motivation is perhaps a less obvious goal, nor is it easy to identify. However, moving from a more cognitive place of attaining or achieving something through purposeful action, I envision motivation to be an embodied experience of joy or enjoyment, and of our natural effort to obtain more of it. A structured, or multi-step, or multi-sensory art experience is meaningless if it does not bring the artist joy. When a person engages in an enjoyable activity, it is highly likely that they will reengage, as it is felt as something fun and worthwhile. Fostering joy in life is an often overlooked therapeutic goal, and yet human beings intrinsically seek joy.

I would argue that most, if not all, of the case vignettes you have thus far read in this book are, in part, stories of how the joy of making art or participating in an arts group was motivation for continuation of engagement. Marcia spoke about this directly in chapter 2, where she connected how her wish to make art motivated her to overcome, at least temporarily, extreme fatigue. Rose also found enough joy in art-making that it moved her to work with her left hand when her dominant right hand was immobile for a time.

Therapeutic Space and Process

Art therapists are accustomed to making the best of less than ideal spaces for art-making. However, there are some basic requirements and steps that are essential for comfort and safety, in particular for those with dementia. These include setting up, assisting, attuning, and pacing.

Setting Up

Accessibility is paramount. Accessibility exists on several levels, from a person learning of the program in the first place, to their ability to get there, pay for it (if there is a fee), and be able to participate without restriction within the space. There needs to be ample room for walkers and wheelchairs, with space on either side so one-on-one work can take place with the therapist/facilitator when needed. Ideally, the space will be designated for art-making only; however, common areas such as dining rooms are often where therapeutic and recreational activities take place. Still, efforts need to be made to ensure the space is free from external noise, intrusion from curious staff, etc. The work tables should be stable, with smooth tops and a strong source of light, such as overhead lighting or a combination of natural and interior light. The art media must be nontoxic and safe to handle, as determined by the art therapist. Food and drinks should be removed so as not to be confused with art supplies. Food items should not be given as art materials without careful consideration of cultural implications as well as safety. For example, would it be viewed as wasteful to use life-sustaining food to make art? Will there be confusion about eating the food rather than using it as art media? Lastly, a small staff-to-participant ratio ensures that one-on-one work (ideally) can help to support those who need more direction.

Assisting

In many circumstances, elders with dementia need individual attention to engage in the art-making. Though an introduction to the use of materials and the plan for the session is sufficient for some, often a more tailored approach is needed. For example, Sondra needed someone to show her what her art materials would do, right in front of her. Sam simply needed a helper to walk him through the steps one or two at a time. Elaine, however, understood the concept better when a helper held her hand as she grasped the brush or pencil, and moved her hand across the paper. This was enough for her to make the connection between the movement of her hand and arm and the creation of the artwork. In general, this work requires being in close physical proximity to the clients, assisting them with the technical aspects of putting paint on the brush or cutting out a shape in paper, etc. This might also require reorienting the clients when needed, or gently encouraging them when they become confused or distracted. Much communication between therapist and client is nonverbal, and so the therapist must pay close attention to body language, shift in mood, or facial expression, as often clients might not be able to express themselves sufficiently through words. As described in chapter 5, this type of assistance is considered the purview of the art therapist's third hand, and as such, it is important that, with whatever assistance is given, the therapist act in the service of the client.

Attuning

Art therapy can help foster image communication and serve as a means of connecting with others. In this way, art therapists explore how to adapt art therapy tools and techniques to work with people who struggle with memory loss and limited communication ability. In their work, art therapists enable people with dementia to discover their own ideas, emotions, and life experiences. While we teach art methods to raise their level of mastery over creative expression, the focus is primarily on fostering feelings of purpose, social connectivity, and self-esteem – variables that are of paramount importance for older peoples' health and well-being. Although these kinds of changes are hard to assess, they are sometimes observed in the subtle ways an individual extends their variety of speech, takes more risk in their artwork, or develops personal links with others in the community. The changes are sometimes deeper. In any event, with the art therapist's gentle encouragement, the older person and the art therapist can engage in a gentle dance of self-expression.

For example, I observed Elana's restlessness before a session began. She was shifting her weight in her wheelchair, with her head twisting back and forth as if looking for something. She repeatedly asked her caregiver the whereabouts of her purse. It seemed to me that she was uncomfortable and anxious. Once I gave the introduction for the session and conducted a demonstration on how to use the materials, I focused my attention on Elana, working at her side, guiding her as she moved through the steps of dipping the paintbrush into water, then paint, then pulling it across the paper. Elena's body relaxed into her chair, her gaze settled in concentration onto her artwork. She smiled as she added more colors to her work. She told me she was painting a garden.

Her body language and demeanor had changed since her arrival in the group, and remained that way throughout the day, as reported by the program director. To me, her calm focus indicated increased comfort and enjoyment that was made possible because of adjustments to help her regain her sense of control.

Pacing

Creative arts therapists encourage freedom of expression within a safe, organizing structure. The therapeutic relationship is fostered by person-centered interactions, paying close attention to embodied, nonverbal communication such as the pacing and pauses in action, efforts to communicate, and modifying pace and type of communication; for example, slowing down speech, movement, and response time to allow time for language and emotional processing. The Iso Principle, used as a method in music therapy to induce a change in mood, sets as the prerequisite that patient's mental tempo has to correlate with the sound-music tempo expressed by the therapist (Benenzon, 2007; Heiderscheit & Madson, 2015). This method of working toward the convergence of divergent paces can be generalized to the development of a new quality in a human relationship, similar to Kossak's (2015) description of attunement with oneself and client in the therapeutic relationship.

Kossak (2015) describes how attunement deepens a therapist's empathy with their client: The therapist first grounds themself by attuning to their own internal rhythm, breath, body, and emotional state and is then able to be more open and aware of the client. It is important for the therapist to be attuned to their own inner world, so that they can be attuned to others. Similarly, in his theory of multiple intelligences, Howard Gardner (2006) describes interpersonal intelligence as a person's knowledge of their internal world and ability to use it for self-understanding and self-expression.

One of the biggest challenges that students face when beginning work with older people with dementia is learning how to slow down to the pace of their client. While the life of a younger person is often driven by schedules, verbal communication, and multiple roles and responsibilities, much of that fades for an older person with dementia. The simple question/answer paradigm that we are accustomed to in daily conversation does not follow the same pattern when communicating with some people with memory loss. When asked a question, that person might need additional time to reply, if at all. However, by paying attention to nonverbal forms of communication such as facial expression, small adjustments to body position, or hand movements can yield clues to the preference or comfort of that person. So, it is important for the carer to adjust their expectation of a quick, verbal response to one that requires patience and focused attention by the carer. Thus, slowing down, pausing, giving the artist time to adjust, and allowing them to do as much as possible without assistance makes it possible to understand the artist's emotional and nonverbal reactions. Likewise, the carer should speak and move more slowly to better align with the pace of the client.

Jacob

A fastidiously dressed man, Jacob had advanced Alzheimer's disease. Jacob was a chemist and accomplished pianist. When we first met, he engaged with me in conversation using single words or brief phrases. Jacob was not interested in making art, no matter what art materials or idea was presented to him. Over time, however, I realized that Jacob needed a particular kind of assistance/support. As was the case with most others there, once we discovered the adaptation or support unique to that person, engagement soared. Jacob would not paint on his own. But when prompted, "Jacob, which color would you like to use?" he announced his choice of color. I then gave him the brush, he dipped it in the corresponding paint, then brushed on a stroke or two of that color, and then stopped. Sometimes, I dipped the brush and gave it to him. When he was done making the strokes, he gave the brush to me, I cleaned it, and then asked him his choice for the next color, and the process repeated until he indicated that he was finished by putting down the brush or closing his eyes. Sometimes, while I was working with other people and he was sitting alone, Jacob would tap his brush on the edge of the table while humming, splattering flecks of paint onto his painting. While I never knew if this was deliberate, it was a joyful surprise how his love for music appeared in his paintings. Rhythmic/repetitive/brush strokes seemed a way for Jacob to engage in the fluid process of painting while maintaining control, for example, *Rhythmic Strokes* (Figure 9.3[1] Rhythmic Strokes).

Figure 9.3 Rhythmic Strokes.

Figure 9.4 Framed Brush Strokes.

While discipline might have been an important aspect of his identity as a scientist and musician, it could also have been a way for him to cope with living in a world distorted by dementia.

Six years later, his functioning declined, and he no longer used words to express himself. Comparing his works over the years, I noticed how the rhythmic precision of his brushwork loosened, as in *Framed Strokes* (Figure 9.4 Framed Brush Strokes). Though he continued in the same style of painting, his colors became muddier as they mixed together unintentionally. The shifts in his artwork reflected the change in his cognitive and physical functioning. However, the rhythmic method by which he painted, and the dance between Jacob and me, the art therapist, did not change. Merely looking at his work does not reveal the unique interaction that supported the art-making process. When I see his work, I see Jacob as he was then. His personality, life experience, and our relationship were richly expressed in those paintings.

Fear and Resistance

Bayles and Orland (1993) identify multiple ways in which setting out to make art is a fear-invoking exercise. There are risks of perceived failure, self-criticism, and more. Committing brush to canvas or pencil to paper is no small endeavor. Our marks are visual expressions of ourselves. I so often hear fellow clinicians saying that their patient or client is "resistant" when they don't want to make art. In my field of mental health, where "compliance" is the ideal, "resistant" is a four-letter word. With so much on the line in making art – expectations, anticipation, risk and fear – much of which we carry with us from our early lives, it is no wonder that our clients might be "resistant" to our invitation to make art!

Before we can ask another person to take such a risk, we have to have taken it ourselves and not only be familiar with the uncomfortable feeling but have developed strategies to overcome fear. Only then can we draw from our own experience to empathize with our client's trepidation and accompany them on their journey. I am learning how to kayak in white-water. I have a healthy amount of fear each time I venture to a pushy river. Do I have the skill to safely paddle this river? As a novice, there are some rivers that I can safely paddle. There are plenty that would be foolish for me to run until I become more skilled and confident. Paddling a river with rapids too advanced for my skill set would not only scare me to near death, but it would also be dangerous, and I would be at risk of getting injured and possibly wanting to quit the sport altogether, not to mention en-dangering my companions. The same risk-to-readiness ratio is vital in approaching art therapy work with anyone. I find this especially true for our older clients and those with dementia in particular. Already faced with micro and macro slights of perceived incompetence by a society that values older people and those with disability as less-than, it is essential that we have adequately "set the stage" for an experience in which the participant can feel they were successful.

As I mentioned earlier, with every encounter I aim to make art-making accessible. Part of this is to redefine what is considered art, framing it as "expression" or "mark making." Many people have only associations to museum-quality art or criticism they received as a child in art class. I work tirelessly to remove the judgment aspect of art-making, replacing it with the belief that any and all marks of visual expression are meaningful and worthwhile. And yet, aesthetic judgment and expectation persist. That is why I aim to build in aesthetic success in each art experience. My hope is that however brief or invested the art-making is, the outcome can be appreciated both aesthetically and conceptually.

Facilitating Success

How do I know what will make my client feel successful? First, I must get to know them: Who is this person in front of me? In some cases, I might have the luxury of reading background information about them from a case file. But in many cases, it is up to me to learn about them. I do this through a complex process of informally assessing their likes and dislikes, their abilities and challenges, and many other aspects of their personality through careful observation. If I am lucky, I will learn about the story of their life, not just the person before me in the present day. In that way, I can draw from their experiences as I devise a plan that might interest them.

Kontos (2005) explains the importance of promoting embodied selfhood in work with people who have dementia. The gist of this notion is that a person is a cumulation of their life and that they embody their life experiences. For example, a person who worked as an industrial designer but now lives with dementia might retain a high level of skill drawing or spatial awareness but not be able to remember where he is or the name of his caregiver. Or a woman who had worked as a lawyer, which requires superior verbal skills, retains a convincing verbal façade that masks her forgetfulness and inability to balance her checkbook or turn off the stove when she is finished cooking. These are extreme examples, but they illustrate how qualities, skills, habits, and preferences from a person's life appear in various ways throughout their life. As a carer of that person, I need to understand how that person's behavior is an embodiment of their cumulative life experience. Body language, the artwork, the art-making process, and more are all ways in which a person expresses their embodiment. And that person must be accepted as they are, even when the means of expression seems problematic and in conflict with the range of acceptable behavior.

Often, I find myself working with people I do not know. At this first meeting, I am simultaneously assessing participants and offering a therapeutic art encounter. In these situations, I want to ensure that my offering is accessible to all. I therefore choose a structured art experience that can be scaled along a continuum of simplicity and complexity, so that each participant experiences success in some way. This is important for a first art therapy experience, especially where a person is making decisions about whether or not art therapy is for them. Even more, people who might already feel disempowered will benefit from an experience in which they feel successful and empowered.

Collage Set Up (Figure 9.5 Collage Set Up) is an example of an art therapy encounter that can easily be scaled and experienced as successful. In the case of this session, I was meeting a group of older people for the first time. I knew that they all were living in a community residence. I did not know anything else, such as if any of them had cognitive loss or physical limitations or if any were coping with symptoms from trauma, among many other possibilities. This "safe" art therapy experience could work with people with and without cognitive impairment. The non-subjective media and prompt were unlikely to trigger a trauma response, and should a person have physical challenges, the materials and tools could easily be adapted.

Ahead of time, I precut many different shapes out of translucent tissue paper, which were spread across the middle of the table for easy access. I mixed water and glue ahead of time and placed them in large containers

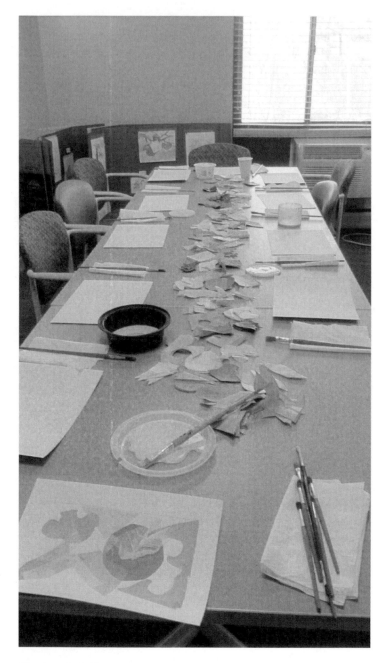

Figure 9.5 Collage Set Up.

between participants. Each place setting had a heavy piece of watercolor paper, a paintbrush, and a paper towel. The idea was to make a collage by layering the tissue paper adhered with glue. The layered tissue paper lends to a beautiful blending of colors, which can be a delightful surprise. The base paper can withstand many layers of paint and glue, thus making it ideal for those artists who wished to fill the frame with complex tissue paper layers, yielding a range of colors and shapes, and forming a sophisticated composition. At the same time, even a simple addition of one or a few pieces of tissue paper to the base paper is an expression of color and shape. Minimalist work is wonderful! The watered-down glue in containers makes application easier than using glue straight from the bottle. Using a paintbrush allows the glue to be applied with more accuracy and keeps hands from getting covered in sticky glue. For those who might not be able to hold a paintbrush, the art therapist can provide assistance by adding glue to shapes that are carefully placed by the participant. Other adaptations can also be made … art therapists are very creative in this way! The simplicity of this media and task makes it accessible for most people. At the same time, for those who are able, the materials can be manipulated in more intricate ways to create complex, detailed, or layered compositions and palettes of color. As there are few restrictions, the experience opens up the possibility of symbolic connection, where the artist can imbue meaning or a story through this media. Similar types of encounters can be offered with other media. For example, semi-moist watercolor paint, with a good range from translucent to opaque, can be especially effective, depending on the amount of water used. Nontoxic and easy to clean and store, the fluidity of these paints supports creative expression with unexpected results and delightful surprises.

The empathic flexibility needed to achieve a successful outcome may appear in numerous ways. While the permutations of what this actually looks like in practice is endless and everchanging, unique to each pairing or group, these are some basic concepts that are particularly relevant when working with people whose functioning might be challenged by circumstances such as cognitive or physical loss that appears in conditions such as dementia, arthritis, macular degeneration, aphasia, etc. They might also be managing social or emotional changes, for example, loneliness, social isolation, or depression.

Three Phases of Group for Dementia

As discussed in chapter 7, the art therapy session is divided into three parts. The first part of the group is used to introduce members or become re-acquainted with one another, and set up and introduce the art materials. This will almost always include giving a brief demonstration of how to use the art materials and what the artwork might look like. So often, participants cannot hear all that is being said, and those with dementia might not understand verbal instructions. I have found that visual demonstration, followed by one-on-one instruction as needed is the most effective way to begin a session of art-making.

The second, and longest, part of the group is for art-making. Participants might need varying degrees of assistance, from reminders about the task at hand to hands-on help manipulating the art media. It is nearly impossible to be a sole group leader in a group of four or more people with advanced dementia, as there are extensive needs to ensure physical safety, emotional containment, redirection, one-on-one instruction, and at the same time, group leadership. Gathering a cadre of helping hands makes the experience the most effective and enjoyable for all.

At the end of the "making" art period, it is vital to close the group with a celebration of the artwork. With the work ideally hung on a wall or at least displayed on the table or held up one by one by me or the artist, each person has the opportunity to introduce their work and then welcome comments from others. Although the discussion might not be linear, thoughts shared by the group are key ingredients to creating a sense of community. Having concrete artwork to present that represents their presence in the group, the artists are recognized by their peers with visual as well as verbal sharing. Sometimes, simply asking the group to offer a title for each work is enough to engage members and stimulate interest. Focusing on the expression of the artwork rather than its theme is most important. In this way, the pressure is removed from interpreting a picture's meaning, which might not be discernible. For example, when the group was asked to give their thoughts about a work, the following comments were offered:

- Bob – "Completely different colors that blend quite well."
- Miranda – "I don't know anything about this one."
- Joe – "Redundancy is helpful to this underground group. I don't comment on my art. I'm suspicious of anyone who does."

Viewing the work sparked conversation among artists that focused on the artwork and each other.

Sometimes, just moments after finishing their work, participants may forget they've made it. Nevertheless, looking at the work this way unites the group, focuses attention on their achievements, and enables a sense of belonging. One day, I experienced a particularly touching moment. Anne, a 102-year-old woman who was sad about her memory loss, shared amazement and joy at her artwork after a student intern verified that the work was, in fact, hers. Anne frequently disregarded and depreciated herself and her work. Her joy upon recognizing her artwork sparked an enthusiastic reaction from other artists, two of whom rarely spoke and a third who applauded her. Anne then said, "If I can do that, maybe I haven't lost all of my mind."

Structured Arts Engagement

Open art sessions offer the largest amount of freedom, which for some participants is the approach that yields the greatest enjoyment and benefit. However, for those with significant cognitive decline, structured art engagement helps a person with dementia engage more fully than if left to the wide range of choice in an open session. Structured art engagement can reduce the feeling of overwhelm or confusion when faced with too many choices. Keeping in mind the aim of fostering connection, communication, and joy, arts engagement activities can be broken into smaller components. The following sections outline how freedom can be achieved through structure, multi-step processes, and sensory stimulation.

Freedom Within Structure

Generally, in a person-centered art therapy program for people with dementia, I try to encourage freedom of expression by creating a safe, organized, and structured session. This includes choosing safe art materials and processes that support success at each turn. I offer elders art materials that are safe and easy to use, and I usually limit the selection so they are not overwhelmed by choices. While the aim is to give as much freedom as possible, it is essential to offer pre-determined art materials that are prepared and set up ahead of time. In that way, decisions that can potentially be distracting or overwhelming to the person with dementia, such as selecting materials, can be minimized. With the art engagement planned ahead of time, the participant can simply interact with the media. For some, simplification of this set up can be frustrating, and thus should be adjusted accordingly. However, for many with significant cognitive decline, this structured art activity gives space for play and freedom to experiment. In the spirit of this freedom, it is important that the therapist or teaching artist accepts all forms of art-making, including those made with fingers, paper scraps, etc. In this way, participants should be offered materials that are safe and easy to use, and with limited selection, not too overwhelming. For example, semi-moist watercolor paints can be offered, along with good quality paper and brushes that can stand up to excessive pressure and water. Using a rectangular or circular outline on the paper to serve as a "frame" often helps to orient and focus the clients.

Structured art therapy activities can take as many forms as artists can imagine them. Some of the structures that I have found to be successful are discussed below, incorporating multi-sensory elements into the art-making process, as well as multi-step processes.

Multi-Step, Multi-Sensory

I have learned that offering an art-making experience that entails a multi-step process is more likely to retain the attention of someone with dementia, and allow for a more layered, complex art-making process. Abstract thinking is required to envision an idea and then execute it through visual media. However, when a person's capacity for abstract thinking diminishes, following a set of instructions can be a way to support functioning, until that also becomes very difficult, if not possible. Thus, in my work with people who have advanced stages of dementia, I have found that offering one step at a time is the most effective approach to maintaining the pace of communication required by the elder's capacity.

Multi-sensory approaches can also be used, for example, presenting items that could be smelled and touched, evoking emotion and memories, such as flowers, shells, oranges, and pinecones, followed by an art-making session. Art-making after multi-sensory stimulation often increases the elder's organization, motivation, and overall enthusiasm for the experience. It can be intimidating to be presented with art materials. What to do with them? Most of us aren't immediately drawn to exploring their potential. However, smell, sound, and touch can evoke an immediate, visceral response, which are particularly valuable attributes available to those with even the most advanced dementia.

One simple yet highly effective approach is to incorporate flowers into a session. Rather than the more traditional approach to placing a bouquet in the center of the table and painting it, individual stems are given to participants to see, touch and smell. This multi-step, multi-sensory hands-on interaction creates a structured experience which lends itself to connection with memories, paint color, and texture. Participants then are better able to translate their sensory experience to painting, prompting a deeper connection with the flowers, paint, and overall group experience. Beginning with multi-step, multi-sensory activities can increase motivation, engagement, and enthusiasm for making art. Bringing texture, smell, and sound into art-making can help artists to have a deeper connection with their memory and feelings, allowing visual expression to be more accessible.

Sunflower Series (Figure 9.6 Sunflower Series) illustrates a group of sunflower paintings that were created with the above process. Sunflowers don't have a prominent smell; however, their large, bright flower commands attention, and their beefy stalk has discernible thickness and texture. Sunflowers have a presence, whether they are placed in a vase in the center of the table or held by hand. A bouquet of sunflowers was presented to the group, first placed in a vase to be observed and admired as well as spark conversation. Artist participants' attention was noticeably elevated and interest piqued as the group focused their attention on the colorful floral presence in front of them. From there, each person held a sunflower stalk and was encouraged to notice its smell, weight, texture, temperature, and anything else. Some were unable to verbally articulate their exploration; however, hands moved more quickly and purposefully up and down the stalk and petal, eyes bright, and a more engaged posture, sitting straighter in their chairs. The time dedicated to

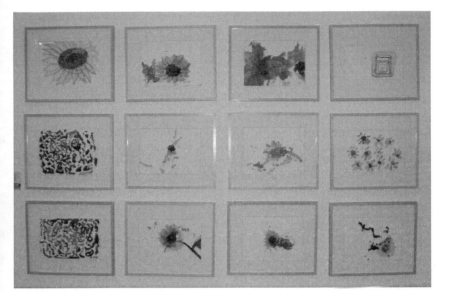

Figure 9.6 Sunflower Series.

this exploration generated noticeable interest in the subject matter. As the participants were given space and time to explore, their interest in the activity increased. When offered art materials to express their experience of the sunflowers, participants transitioned more quickly than usual, making connections between the colors in the flower and in the palette. I believe that the step of holding and engaging tactically with the flower was an important step in attuning the clients to the activity and the subject matter, as well as giving them time to take in the sensory experience and experience enjoyment.

Music

As an accompaniment in an art therapy session, music can be very useful in eliciting participants' memories and their current emotional states. Various styles and genres can inspire participants to paint in different ways. Music can influence all elements of the group, such as painting styles, brushstrokes, colors, ability to focus, interaction among group members, thematic artistic content, topics of conversation, and the general mood of the session. Paul, a man with advanced dementia, frequently adjusted his way of making art according to the music played. When we played upbeat jazz, his colors would become bolder. His art also became more lyrical, with lighter, more fluid colors that appeared to mimic the playful, classical music being played. Often using repetitive brush strokes that would ultimately wear a hole in the paper, music lightened Paul's pressure on his brush. Instead, music seemed to lift his hand – skating more gently across the entirety of the paper canvas. We found that softer music encouraged a calmer painting process that was more of an individualistic focus with less group interaction. For Paul, the purposeful incorporation of music stimulated his creative expression in visual media. Music activated him and was instrumental in motivating and increasing his self-expression.

Concluding Thoughts

Dementia is a cruel disease, stripping a person of their functioning and personality. Families lose their loved one long before they have actually died, as they slowly fade and change. And yet, as dementia chips away at the social façade that has been carefully crafted for decades, the essence of that person is exposed and unfiltered. That essence is ripe for creative expression, as filters and rules are not necessary for art to flourish. Though in them loss is evident, so is life. My experience working side by side with some of the people introduced in this chapter, wordless, but not in silence, has been among the most joyful moments in my life.

Note

1 This image has been redrawn by the author due to poor photographic quality of the original work.

References

Abraham, R. (2005). *When words have lost their meaning: Alzheimer's patients communicate through art.* Westport, CT: Praeger Publishers/Greenwood Publishing Group.

American Psychiatric Association. (2011). *Practice guideline for the treatment of patients with Alzheimer's disease and other dementias.* Arlington, VA: American Psychiatric Association.

Bayles, D., & Orland, T. (1993). *Art and fear: Observations on the perils (and rewards) of artmaking.* Image Continuum Press.

Benenzon, R. O. (2007). The Benenzon Model. *Nordic Journal of Music Therapy, 16*(2), 148.

Dugmore, O., Orrell, M., & Spector, A. (2015). Qualitative studies of psychosocial interventions for dementia: A systematic review. *Aging & Mental Health, 19*(11), 955–967. https://doi-org.ezproxyles.flo.org/10.1080/13607863.2015.1011079

Gardner, H. (2006). *Multiple intelligences: New horizons* (Completely rev. and updated). New York: Basic Books.

Gonen, J., & Soroker, N. (2000). Art therapy in stroke rehabilitation: A model of short-term group treatment. *The Arts in Psychotherapy, 27*(1), 41–50.

Hattori, H., Hattori, C., Hokao, C., Mizushima, K., & Mase, T. (2011). Controlled study on the cognitive and psychological effect of coloring and drawing in mild Alzheimer's disease patients. *Geriatrics & Gerontology International, 11*, 431–437.

Heiderscheit, A., & Madson, A. (2015). Use of the iso principle as a central method in mood management: A music psychotherapy clinical case study. *Music Therapy Perspectives, 33*(1), 45.

Horovitz, E. (2005). *Art therapy as witness: A sacred guide.* Springfield, IL: Charles C. Thomas Publisher.

Hunter, A., Keady, J., Casey, D., Grealish, A., & Murphy, K. (2016). Psychosocial intervention use in long-stay dementia care: A classic grounded theory. *Qualitative Health Research, 26*(14), 2024–2034.

Kim, S., Kim, M., Lee, J., & Chun, S. (2008). Art therapy outcomes in the rehabilitation treatment of a stroke patient: A case report. *Art Therapy: Journal of the American Art Therapy Association, 25*(3), 129–133.

Kontos, P. C. (2005). Embodied selfhood in Alzheimer's disease: Rethinking person-centred care. *Dementia, 4*, 553.

Kontos, P., & Grigorovich, A. (2018a). Rethinking musicality in dementia as embodied and relational. *Journal of Aging Studies, 45*, 39–48. https://doi-org.ezproxyles.flo.org/10.1016/j.jaging.2018.01.006

Kontos, P., & Grigorovich, A. (2018b). Integrating citizenship, embodiment, and relationality: Toward a reconceptualization of dance and dementia in long-term care. *Journal of Law, Medicine & Ethics, 46*(3), 717–723. https://doi-org.ezproxyles.flo.org/10.1177/1073110518804233

Kossak, M. (2015). *Attunement in expressive arts therapy: Toward an understanding of embodied empathy.* Springfield, IL: Charles C. Thomas Publisher, Ltd.

Lee, R., Wong, J., Shoon, W. L., Gandhi, M., Lei, F., Kua, E. H., Rawtaer, I., & Mahendran, R. (2019). Art therapy for the prevention of cognitive decline. *The Arts in Psychotherapy, 64*, 20–25.

Logsdon, R. G., & Teri, L. (2018). Quality of life in dementia: Conceptualization, measurement, and psychosocial treatment implications. In *APA handbook of dementia* (pp. 237–248). American Psychological Association. https://doi-org.ezproxyles.flo.org/10.1037/0000076–012

Mimica, N., & Dubravka K. (2011). Art therapy may be beneficial for reducing stress-related behaviours in people with dementia--case report. *Psychiatria Danubina, 23*(1), 125–128.

Rusted, J., Sheppard, L., & Waller, D. (2006). Therapy for older people with dementia. *Group Analysis, 4*(39), 517–536.

Sacchett, C., Byng, S., Marshall, J., & Pound, C. (1999). Drawing together: Evaluation of a therapy programme for severe aphasia. *International Journal of Language and Communication Disorders, 34*(3), 265–289.

Schall, A., Haberstroh, J., & Pantel, J. (2015). Time series analysis of individual music therapy in dementia: Effects on communication behavior and emotional well-being. *GeroPsych: The Journal of Gerontopsychology and Geriatric Psychiatry, 28*(3), 113–122. https://doi-org.ezproxyles.flo.org/10.1024/1662–9647/a000123

Stephenson, R. C. (2015). Color my words--How art therapy creates new pathways of communication. In L. Cardoza (Ed.), *Communication and aging: Creative approaches to improving the quality of life* (pp. 247–267). San Diego, CA: Plural Publishing, Inc.

Symons, J., Clark, H., Williams, K., Hansen, E., & Orpin, P. (2011). Visual art in physical rehabilitation: Experience of people with neurological conditions. *British Journal of Occupational Therapy*, *74*(1), 44–52.

Teri, L., McKenzie, G., & LaFazia, D. (2005). Psychosocial treatment of depression in older adults with dementia. *Clinical Psychology: Science and Practice*, *12*, 303–316.

Zaidel, D. W. (2013). Biological and neuronal underpinnings of creativity in the arts. In O. Vartanian, A. S. Bristol, & J. C. Kaufman (Eds.), *Neuroscience of Creativity* (pp. 133–148). Cambridge, MA: MIT Press.

Zhao, J., Li, H., Lin, R., Wei, Y., & Yang, A. (2019). Effects of creative expression therapy for older adults with mild cognitive impairment at risk of Alzheimer's disease: A randomized controlled clinical trial. *Clinical Interventions in Aging*, *13*, 1313–1320. doi.org/10.2147/CIA.S161861

Epilogue

The Covid-19 pandemic lingers on at the time this book is going to press. The stories and approaches presented here are from a pre-pandemic time when we gathered in person. Elder artists shared art materials, and the sensory experience of them, such as the smell of clay, or the sound of several people drawing vigorously at once. Art therapists' intuitive and relational sensibilities could be fully utilized in this environment, noticing nuanced facial and body expression, for example. The importance of place and safe space was physical as well as emotional. Traveling from one's residence to the location of art making was a notable transitional process of arriving and departing that allowed the artist to anticipate and then process their participation.

Many if not most programs have now either suspended service, significantly reduced it, or moved to an online format. At the time of writing this epilogue, therapists and clients alike have had close to a year to adjust to Zoom therapy. What initially seemed like a risky experiment has now become part of everyday life. Who is to say what will happen to these programs when the pandemic finally ends? Likely, some of the adaptations will remain, as some of them, as it turns out, have their benefits.

The Lenox Hill CARE program is a remarkable example of a successful transition to online programming for their members. As discussed at length in this book, connection is vital to a person's well-being. Despite the loss of in-person connection among members of the CARE community of elders with dementia, their caregivers, family members, and the program staff, students, and volunteers, the daily online program has been a lifeline for all of them. Some of the benefits of this format, as noted by the program director Elizabeth Hartowicz (personal communication, November 19, 2020), have been unexpected. For example, the ability to participate from the comfort of home eliminates the stress of preparing oneself to leave for the day and coping with traffic congestion, delays, and other distractions that occur when participants attend in person. Their home environment is predictable, comfortable, and better suited to meet their changing needs throughout the day.

The energy among a group of people gathered in a room in undeniable. However, the sound of multiple conversations can be distracting, and it might be difficult to hear or see the person speaking at the other end of the room. Instead, the computer screen brings the program close up. The facsimile of sound and image, although somewhat distorted, can be far more accessible to some than what they might experience in person. The assistance needed by the caregivers to operate the technology is essential, and without it, participation is at risk. However, Elizabeth reports that the additional effort of caregivers helping to facilitate the receiving end of the program has created a deeper connection between the caregiver and elder, plus a broader support network with other caregivers.

It is hard to imagine at the moment that a program like CARE would not return in person. And yet, there are some real benefits to the online delivery model that could not have been anticipated. There will be opportunities to integrate the ideas in this book with new approaches to care that arose as we responded and adapted to the pandemic with immense creativity.

The pandemic has altered our lives and will no doubt leave a lasting impact on the healthcare system. It is my sincere hope that the sacrifices and losses endured during the pandemic will yield a better and more equitable world, with a health care system that truly serves each and every person.

Index